KEY GOVERNMENT REPORTS

VOLUME 26

HEALTH CARE – JUNE 2019

KEY GOVERNMENT REPORTS

Additional books and e-books in this series can be found on Nova's website under the Series tab.

KEY GOVERNMENT REPORTS

VOLUME 26

HEALTH CARE – JUNE 2019

ERNEST CLARK
EDITOR

snova
New York

NOTICE TO THE READER

Additional color graphics may be available in the e-book version of this book.

Library of Congress Cataloging-in-Publication Data

ISBN: 978-1-53616-568-5

Published by Nova Science Publishers, Inc. † New York

CONTENTS

PREFACE

This book is a comprehensive compilation of all reports, testimony, correspondence and other publications issued by the GAO (Government Accountability Office) during the month of June, grouped according to the topic: Health Care.

Chapter 1 - Since 2009, GAO has produced a body of work on the Black Lung Benefits Program. In 2018, for instance, GAO reported that the Trust Fund, which pays benefits to certain coal miners, faced financial challenges due, in part, to the coal tax rate decrease that took effect in 2019 and declining coal production. Trust Fund finances could be further strained by coal mine operator bankruptcies, as they can lead to benefit liabilities being transferred to the Trust Fund. This chapter describes Trust Fund finances through 2050 and provides preliminary observations from ongoing work for this committee regarding the Department of Labor's (DOL) oversight of coal mine operator insurance. To describe Trust Fund finances, in its 2018 report GAO developed simulations through 2050 based on various assumptions related to future coal production and the number of future black lung beneficiaries. To develop preliminary observations from its ongoing work, GAO analyzed DOL documentation and data on black lung beneficiaries and coal mine operators. GAO also reviewed relevant federal laws, regulations, policies, and guidance and interviewed DOL officials, insurance carriers, and coal mine operators, among others.

Chapter 2 - Specialty care referrals are a key component of care coordination for TRICARE Prime beneficiaries. Each Prime beneficiary is assigned to a primary care manager either at an MTF or within the civilian provider network. Primary care managers are responsible for overseeing all aspects of their patients' care, which includes making referrals for specialty care when needed. The National Defense Authorization Act for Fiscal Year 2017 included a provision for GAO to examine care coordination within and between the direct and purchased care systems. Among other objectives, this chapter examines the extent to which the referral management process facilitates the coordination of primary and specialty care for TRICARE Prime beneficiaries. GAO examined relevant policies; analyzed current referral data from five MTFs it visited, selected for variety in military service, geographic location, and numbers of referrals; and interviewed officials with DHA and the military services. GAO also discussed the implementation of MHS Genesis with officials at DOD and the four MTFs where it has been implemented.

Chapter 3 - VA continues to focus on the use of community care to address challenges with veterans' access to health care services at VA medical facilities. In fiscal year 2019, VA plans to consolidate the Veterans Choice Program and several other community care programs under a single new Veterans Community Care Program. GAO and others have previously reported on past challenges VA has faced regarding the reliability, transparency, and consistency of its budget estimates for health care. GAO was asked to review VA's use of community care and efforts to develop budget estimates for this care. This chapter describes (1) trends in obligations for and utilization of VA's community care programs since fiscal year 2014, (2) how VA develops its community care budget estimate and any subsequent changes made to this estimate, and (3) how VA's actual obligations for community care compared with estimated obligations for fiscal years 2017 and 2018. GAO reviewed actual obligation and utilization data for fiscal years 2014 through 2018, as well as estimated obligations for fiscal years 2019 through 2021. GAO also reviewed available VA documentation on the methods and data used to develop VA's community care budget estimate that informed the President's budget request for fiscal years 2017 through 2019. GAO also interviewed VA officials and contractors responsible for developing these estimates, and OMB staff responsible for the federal budget. VA and OMB reviewed a draft of this chapter. VA's technical comments were incorporated as appropriate.

Chapter 4 - VHA operates one of the nation's largest health care systems with 18 regional networks—VISNs—that manage and oversee 172 medical centers within defined geographic areas. VHA expects to provide care to more than 7 million veterans in fiscal year 2019, and demand for its services is expected to grow over time. GAO was asked to conduct a review of VISNs, including VHA's oversight of VISNs. This chapter examines (1) the extent to which VHA oversees VISNs' management and oversight of medical centers and (2) how VHA oversees VISN staffing. GAO reviewed VHA policies, guidance, and staffing data regarding VISNs. GAO also interviewed officials from VHA, all 18 VISNs, and four medical centers selected for variation in geography, urban or rural location, and complexity.

Chapter 5 - VA provides for care to over 9-million veterans in its health care system, including 172 VAMCs. As veterans' demographics shift, such as by age or gender, their needs for health care and their expectations for how they receive that care may also change. Along with the VA MISSION Act of 2018, which requires VA to assess its facilities for realignment and modernization, these changes could have implications for VA's capital-planning efforts. GAO was asked to review how VA incorporates veterans' changing needs and expectations into facility planning. This chapter examines: (1) VA's efforts to assess trends in veterans' future needs and expectations; (2) VA's efforts to help VAMCs address these changes through facility planning; and (3) how VAMCs use VA's process for identifying facilities' future space needs. GAO surveyed all VAMCs, visited nine VAMCs, reviewed VA's planning documents and data, and interviewed officials from VA and veterans service organizations. GAO's survey response rate was 99 percent.

In: Key Government Reports. Volume 26 ISBN: 978-1-53616-568-5
Editor: Ernest Clark

Chapter 1

Black Lung Benefits Program: Financing and Oversight Challenges Are Adversely Affecting the Trust Fund*

Cindy Brown Barnes

Why GAO Did This Study

Since 2009, GAO has produced a body of work on the Black Lung Benefits Program. In 2018, for instance, GAO reported that the Trust Fund, which pays benefits to certain coal miners, faced financial challenges due, in part, to the coal tax rate decrease that took effect in 2019 and declining coal production. Trust Fund finances could be further strained by coal mine

* This is an edited, reformatted and augmented version of the United States Government Accountability Office Testimony Before the Committee on Education and Labor, Subcommittee on Workforce Protections, House of Representatives, Publication No. GAO-19-622T, dated June 20, 2019.

operator bankruptcies, as they can lead to benefit liabilities being transferred to the Trust Fund.

This testimony describes Trust Fund finances through 2050 and provides preliminary observations from ongoing work for this committee regarding the Department of Labor's (DOL) oversight of coal mine operator insurance.

To describe Trust Fund finances, in its 2018 report GAO developed simulations through 2050 based on various assumptions related to future coal production and the number of future black lung beneficiaries. To develop preliminary observations from its ongoing work, GAO analyzed DOL documentation and data on black lung beneficiaries and coal mine operators. GAO also reviewed relevant federal laws, regulations, policies, and guidance and interviewed DOL officials, insurance carriers, and coal mine operators, among others.

WHAT GAO RECOMMENDS

GAO will be considering recommendations, as appropriate, when ongoing work is finished.

WHAT GAO FOUND

GAO reported in 2018 that Black Lung Disability Trust Fund (Trust Fund) expenditures have consistently exceeded revenue. The Trust Fund borrowed from the Department of the Treasury's (Treasury) general fund and hence from the taxpayer almost every year since 1979, its first complete fiscal year, causing debt and interest to accumulate. Federal law does not limit the amount the Trust Fund may borrow as needed to cover its expenditures. Trust Fund revenue will be further limited by the coal tax rate decrease of about 55 percent that took effect in 2019, and declining coal production, according to GAO's simulation. Specifically, Trust Fund revenue may not be sufficient to cover beneficiary payments and administrative costs, from fiscal years 2020 through 2050. Therefore, the Trust Fund could need to continue borrowing to cover its expenditures—including the repayment of past debt and interest—and the Trust Fund's simulated outstanding debt could exceed $15 billion by 2050 (see figure). However, as GAO reported in 2018, various options, such as adjusting the coal tax and forgiving debt, could improve the Trust Fund's financial position.

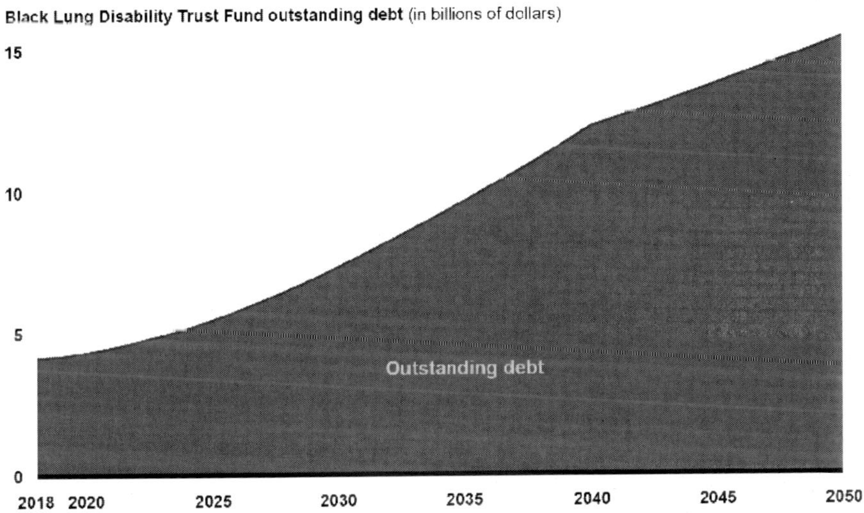

Source: GAO simulation based on data from the Department of Labor and Treasury, the Energy information Administration, and the Office of Management and Budget. | GAO-19-622T.

Trust Fund Simulated Outstanding Debt, Fiscal Years 2018 through 2050.

GAO's preliminary observations indicate that Trust Fund finances will be further strained by coal operator bankruptcies. Since 2014, an estimated black lung benefit liability of over $310 million has been transferred to the Trust Fund from insolvent self-insured coal mine operators, according to DOL data. Federal law generally requires that operators secure their black lung benefit liability. To do so, operators can self-insure if they meet certain DOL conditions. As of June 2019, there are 22 operators that are self-insured and actively mining coal, according to DOL officials. GAO's preliminary analysis indicates that DOL did not regularly review these operators so that it could adjust collateral as needed to protect the Trust Fund. As a result, the amount of collateral DOL required from some of these operators is tens of millions less than their most recent estimated black lung benefit liability.

Chairwoman Adams, Ranking Member Byrne, and Members of the Subcommittee:

I am pleased to be here today to highlight GAO's prior and ongoing work on Black Lung Disability Trust Fund (Trust Fund) solvency, and the Department of Labor's (DOL) oversight of coal mine operator insurance given recent operator bankruptcies.[1]

The Black Lung Benefits Program provides medical and cash assistance to certain coal miners who have been totally disabled due to pneumoconiosis, also known as black lung disease.[2] Their surviving dependents may also receive assistance. Black lung benefits are generally to be paid by liable coal mine operators. However, the Trust Fund pays benefits in certain circumstances including in cases where no responsible mine operator could be identified or when the liable mine operator does not pay. The Trust Fund is financed primarily by a tax on coal produced and sold domestically, which we refer to in this statement as the coal tax.[3]

In 2018, we reported that the Trust Fund faced financial challenges and borrowed about $1.3 billion in fiscal year 2017 from the Department of the Treasury's (Treasury) general fund to cover its expenditures. Beginning in 2019, the rate of the coal tax—the Trust Fund's primary revenue source—decreased by about 55 percent. The Trust Fund may also be affected by declining future coal production, as we reported in 2018. With less revenue from the coal tax, increased federal funding will likely be needed. Under

---

[1] GAO, *Black Lung Benefits Program: Options to Improve Trust Fund Finances*, GAO-18-351 (Washington D.C: May 30, 2018).

[2] Black lung is caused by breathing coal mine dust and the severity of the disease can range from mild—with no noticeable effects on breathing—to advanced disease, which could lead to respiratory failure and death according to the Centers for Disease Control, National Institute of Occupational Safety and Health.

[3] The coal tax is imposed on the sale of all domestic coal with two exceptions: (1) lignite coal and (2) exported coal.

federal law the Trust Fund borrows from Treasury's general fund when necessary to cover its expenditures. Federal law does not limit the amount the Trust Fund may borrow from Treasury's general fund—and hence from the taxpayer—as needed to cover its relevant expenditures. However, various options, such as adjusting the coal tax and forgiving interest or debt, could reduce future borrowing and improve the Trust Fund's financial position (see GAO-18-351).

In my testimony today, I will (1) discuss the future solvency of the Trust Fund given the coal tax rate decrease and declining coal production, and (2) provide preliminary observations based on ongoing work for this committee regarding DOL's oversight of coal mine operator insurance given recent operator bankruptcies.

To address our first objective we drew directly from our 2018 report. In that report we simulated, among other things, how Trust Fund debt may change through 2050 given the coal tax rate decrease and declining coal production.[4] Our simulations were based on various assumptions and simulated Trust Fund revenues and expenditures from fiscal years 2016 through 2050. To develop these simulations, we used actual and projection data from (1) DOL for fiscal years 2015 through 2040; (2) Treasury's Office of Tax Analysis for fiscal years 2011 through 2015; (3) the Department of Energy's Energy Information Administration (EIA) for calendar years 2015 through 2050; and (4) the Office of Management and Budget (OMB) for fiscal year 2017. We ran each simulation multiple times using different sets of assumptions about the number of future black lung beneficiaries and future coal production. Doing so provided a range of estimates about the Trust Fund's future borrowing needs and provided insight on the sensitivity of its overall financial position relative to its revenues and expenditures. In this testimony, as we did in our report, we generally present the results of a moderate set of assumptions for each simulation.[5] We assessed the reliability of the data used to develop our

---

[4] Our simulations began in fiscal year 2016 because 2015 was the last complete fiscal year for which DOL data were available when we began our review. Our simulations extend through fiscal year 2050 as this is the last year of EIA coal production forecast estimates.

[5] [5]For more information on our simulation methodology and the full range of results, see GAO-18-351.

simulations by interviewing knowledgeable agency officials and reviewing relevant supporting documentation describing the inputs and assumptions used, if applicable. We also reviewed DOL, Treasury, EIA, and OMB data for outliers, obvious errors, or missing data. We determined that the data were sufficiently reliable for the purposes of our report.

Our preliminary observations regarding DOL's oversight of coal mine operator insurance given recent operator bankruptcies are based on ongoing work for this committee. In conducting this work, we obtained DOL documentation and data on black lung beneficiaries and coal mine operators. We also reviewed relevant federal laws, regulations, policies, and guidance and interviewed DOL officials, insurance carriers and associations, and coal mine operators, among others.[6]

We conducted the work on which this statement is based in accordance with generally accepted government auditing standards. Those standards require that we plan and perform the audit to obtain sufficient, appropriate evidence to provide a reasonable basis for our findings and conclusions based on our audit objectives. We believe that the evidence obtained provides a reasonable basis for our findings and conclusions based on our audit objectives.

BACKGROUND

Black Lung Benefits

Black lung benefits include both cash assistance and medical benefits. Maximum cash assistance payments ranged from about $660 to $1,320 per month in 2018, depending on a beneficiary's number of dependents.[7]

[6] We did not conduct a legal analysis of the relevant bankruptcy court dockets. Instead, we relied on documentation provided by DOL to describe these bankruptcies.

[7] Benefit rates are set by federal law, which specifies that in the case of total disability, a miner receives 37.5 percent of the monthly pay rate of a federal employee at grade GS-2, step 1. Benefit levels are increased by 50 percent if the miner has one dependent, 75 percent if the miner has two dependents, and 100 percent if the miner has three or more dependents. If state workers' compensation benefits are less than federal black lung benefits, then the

Miners receiving cash assistance are also eligible for medical benefits that cover the treatment of their black lung-related conditions, which may include hospital and nursing care, rehabilitation services, and drug and equipment charges, according to DOL documentation. DOL estimates that the average annual cost for medical treatment in fiscal year 2018 was approximately $9,667 per miner.

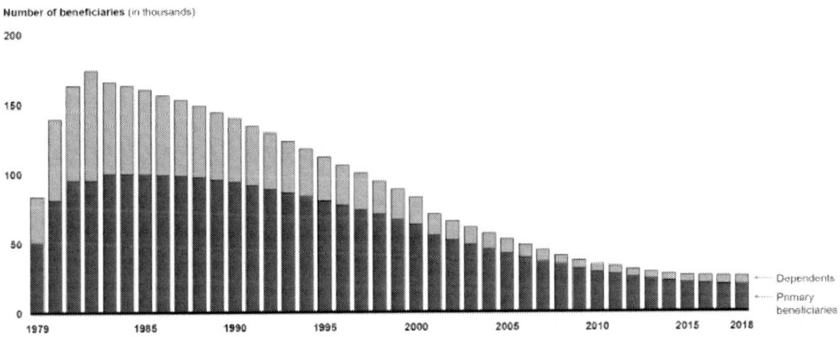

GAO analysis data Departen of Labor data. | GAO-19-622T.

Notes: We excluded certain black lung beneficiaries, which the Department of Labor refers to as Part B beneficiaries, whose awards are generally funded from Treasury's general fund, and not the Trust Fund.

Figure 1. Black Lung Beneficiaries, Fiscal Years 1979 through 2018.

There were about 25,600 total beneficiaries (primary and dependents) receiving black lung benefits during fiscal year 2018 (see figure 1).[8] The number of beneficiaries has decreased over time as a result of declining coal mining employment and an aging beneficiary population, according DOL officials. Black lung beneficiaries could increase in the near term due to the increased occurrence of black lung disease and its most severe form, progressive massive fibrosis, particularly among Appalachian coal miners,

---

federal benefits cover the difference. Social Security Disability Insurance benefits are also reduced for recipients of black lung benefits.

[8] We excluded certain black lung beneficiaries, which DOL refers to as Part B beneficiaries, whose awards are generally funded from Treasury's general fund, and not from the Trust Fund.

according to National Institute for Occupational Safety and Health (NIOSH) officials.[9]

Benefit Adjudication Process

Black lung claims are processed by the Division of Coal Mine Workers' Compensation in the Office of Workers' Compensation Programs (OWCP) within DOL. Contested claims are adjudicated by DOL's Office of Administrative Law Judges (OALJ), which issues decisions that can be appealed to DOL's Benefits Review Board (BRB).[10] Claimants and mine operators may further appeal these agency decisions to the federal courts. If an award is contested, claimants can receive interim benefits, which are generally paid from the Trust Fund according to DOL officials. Final awards are either funded by mine operators—who are identified as the responsible employers of claimants—or the Trust Fund, when responsible employers cannot be identified or do not pay. In fiscal year 2018, black lung claims had an approval rate of about 34 percent, according to DOL data.

In 2009, we reported on the benefits adjudication process and made several recommendations for DOL that could improve miners' ability to pursue claims.[11] An April 2015 DOL Inspector General (IG) report followed up on DOL's progress on our recommendations and found continuing problems and raised new concerns about the black lung claims and appeals process.[12] For instance, the IG reported that OALJ needed to

---

[9] Recent NIOSH studies have found increases in the prevalence of black lung disease among long tenured Appalachian coal miners and have documented hundreds of miners with the most severe form of the disease, progressive massive fibrosis, receiving care at two clinics in Kentucky and Virginia. See D.J. Blackley, L.E. Reynolds, C. Short, R. Carson, E. Storey, C.N. Halldin, A.S. Laney, *Progressive Massive Fibrosis in Coal Miners From 3 Clinics in Virginia,* Journal of the American Medical Association, 319(5):500–501 February 6, 2018; and D.J. Blackley, J.B Crum, C.N. Halldin, E. Storey, A.S. Laney, *Resurgence of Progressive Massive Fibrosis in Coal Miners — Eastern Kentucky, 2016*, Morbidity and Mortality Weekly Report, 65:1385–1389 (December 16, 2016).

[10] For additional information on the black lung claim adjudication process see GAO, *Black Lung Benefits Program: Administrative and Structural Changes Could Improve Miners' Ability to Pursue Claims*. GAO-10-7 (Washington, D.C.: October 30, 2009).

[11] See GAO-10-7.

[12] Office of the Inspector General-Office of Audit, U.S. Department of Labor, Report to the Office of Workers' Compensation Program, Office of Administrative Law Judges, and Benefits Review Board, *Procedural Changes Could Reduce the Time Required to*

address staff shortages, improve communication between its headquarters and district offices, and upgrade the training provided to judges and law clerks.[13] To further expedite claim adjudication, the IG recommended, among other things, that OALJ begin hearing more cases remotely using video or telephone hearings to reduce judges' travel costs and time.[14] In fiscal year 2018, OWCP reported that it took about 335 days on average to issue a decision on a claim. This is an increase from the average of 235 days that OWCP had reported to the DOL IG for fiscal year 2014.[15]

Trust Fund Revenue and Expenditures

Trust Fund revenue is primarily obtained from mine operators through the coal tax. The current coal tax rates, which took effect in 2019, are $0.50 per ton of underground-mined coal and $0.25 per ton of surface-mined coal, up to 2 percent of the sales price. Coal tax revenue is collected from mine operators by Treasury's Internal Revenue Service and then transferred to the Trust Fund where it is then used by DOL to pay black lung benefits and the costs of administering the program.

Trust Fund expenditures include, among other things, black lung benefit payments, certain administrative costs incurred by DOL and Treasury to administer the black lung benefits program, and debt repayments. When necessary for the Trust Fund to make relevant expenditures under federal law, the Trust Fund borrows from the Treasury's general fund. When this occurs, the federal government is

---

Adjudicate Federal Black Lung Benefits Claims, 05-15-001-50-598 (Washington, D.C.: April 9, 2015).

[13] In September 2017, the DOL IG reported that OALJ could reduce its backlog of black lung cases by 21 percent or 28 percent by adding 3 or 6 judges. See Office of the Inspector General-Office of Audit, U.S. Department of Labor, Report to the Office of Administrative Law Judges, *Effect of OALJ Staffing Levels on the Black Lung Case Backlog*, 05-17-003-01-060 (Washington, D.C.: September 27, 2017).

[14] GAO made a related recommendation in 2009 that DOL consider shortening the time required to schedule hearings for black lung cases by examining the feasibility of using video teleconferencing technology to streamline the scheduling of hearings in remote areas, see GAO-10-7.

[15] See Office of the Inspector General-Office of Audit, U.S. Department of Labor, 05-15- 001-50-598.

essentially borrowing from itself—and hence from the taxpayer—to fund its benefit payments and other expenditures.

Trust Fund Borrowing Will Likely Continue to Increase through 2050

As we reported in 2018, Trust Fund expenditures have consistently exceeded revenue. The Trust Fund borrowed from Treasury's general fund almost every year since 1979, its first complete fiscal year.[16] We noted in our 2018 report that Trust Fund borrowing would continue to increase through 2050 due, in part, to the planned coal tax rate decrease of about 55 percent that took effect in 2019 and declining coal production.

We simulated the effects of the tax rate decrease on Trust Fund finances through 2050, and reported the results of a moderate case set of assumptions related to future coal production and prices and the number of new black lung beneficiaries.[17] These simulations were not predictions of what will happen, but rather models of what could happen given certain assumptions.

Our moderate case simulation suggested that Trust Fund revenue may decrease from about $485 million in fiscal year 2018 to about $298 million in fiscal year 2019, due, in part, to the approximate 55 percent decrease in the coal tax rate.[18] Our simulation, which incorporated EIA data on future expected coal production, also showed that annual Trust Fund revenue

---

[16] When necessary for the Trust Fund to make relevant expenditures, funds are appropriated to the Trust Fund as "repayable advances," and then those advances must be repaid with interest to the general fund of the U.S. Treasury. We refer to this process as annual borrowing from Treasury's general fund because, for reporting purposes, we often refer to the total amount of the repayable advances made in a particular fiscal year. According to the Department of the Treasury, the general fund includes assets and liabilities used to finance the daily and long-term operations of the U.S. government as a whole.

[17] Our simulations began in fiscal year 2016 because fiscal year 2015 was the last complete fiscal year for which DOL data were available when we began our review. Our simulations extend through fiscal year 2050 because that is as far as the EIA produces coal production forecasts which we relied on in developing our simulations relative to future coal tax revenue. For more information on our simulation methodology, see GAO-18-351.

[18] The simulated values for Trust Fund revenue and expenditures through 2050 are presented in nominal dollars, meaning they are not adjusted for inflation.

would likely continue to decrease beyond fiscal year 2019 due, in part, to declining coal production. Domestic coal production declined from about 1.2 billion tons in 2008 to about 775 million tons in 2017, according to EIA.[19] Based on these projections, our moderate simulation showed that Trust Fund annual revenue may continue to decrease from about $298 million in fiscal year 2019 to about $197 million in fiscal year 2050.[20]

Future simulated Trust Fund revenue would likely be insufficient to cover combined black lung benefit payments and administrative costs, according to our moderate case simulation. Specifically, revenue may not be sufficient to cover beneficiary payments and administrative costs from fiscal years 2020 through 2050 (see fig. 2). For instance, in fiscal year 2029, simulated benefit payments and administrative costs would likely exceed simulated revenue by about $99 million.[21] These annual deficits could decrease over time to about $4 million by fiscal year 2050 due, in part, to the assumed continued net decline in total black lung beneficiaries.[22]

If Trust Fund spending on benefit payments and administrative costs continues to exceed revenues each year, then the Trust Fund would need to continue borrowing from Treasury's general fund to cover those costs, as well as borrowing to cover debt repayment. Our moderate simulation suggested that the Trust Fund's outstanding debt could increase from about $4.2 billion in fiscal year 2019 to about $15.4 billion in fiscal year 2050 (see figure 3). While our moderate case simulated a $15.4 billion Trust Fund debt in 2050, the amount could vary from about $6 billion to about $27 billion depending, in part, on future coal production and the number of new beneficiaries. Even if the Congress were to completely eliminate black lung benefits as of fiscal year 2019, the Trust Fund's outstanding debt in

---

[19] U.S. Department of Energy, Energy Information Administration: *Annual Coal Report 2017* (Washington, D.C.: November 2018).

[20] These are equivalent to about $290 million and $100 million in 2018 after adjusting for inflation.

[21] This is equivalent to about $78 million in 2018 after adjusting for inflation.

[22] This is equivalent to about $2 million in 2018 after adjusting for inflation.

fiscal year 2050 could still exceed $6.4 billion, according to our simulation.[23]

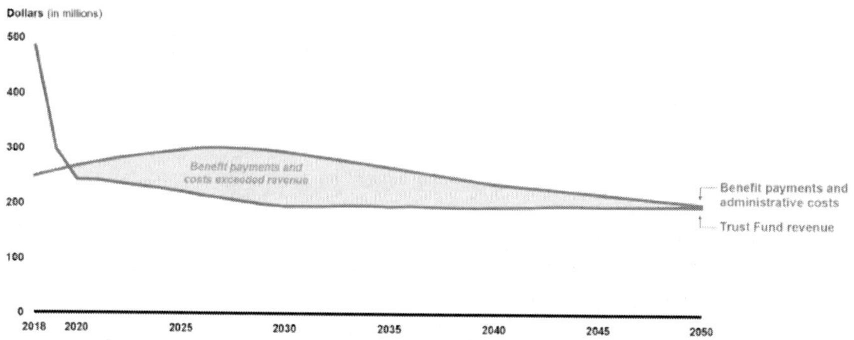

Source: GAO simulation based on data from the Department of Labor and Treasury, the Energy information Administration, and the Office of Management and Budget. | GAO-19-622T.

Notes: Trust Fund revenue and black lung benefit payments and administrative costs are simulated from fiscal years 2018 through 2050 and presented in nominal dollars. Moderate case simulations assumed that future coal production is consistent with the Energy Information Administration's reference case, which generally assumes trend improvement in known technologies, a view of economic and demographic trends that reflects the current central views of economic forecasters and demographers, and that current laws and regulations affecting the energy sector are unchanged through 2050. Moderate case simulations also assumed that future numbers of new black lung beneficiaries evolve over time based on the average growth rate for the period from fiscal years 2003 to 2015. Given the complexities of estimating future coal production and prices and new black lung beneficiaries, our simulations are subject to considerable uncertainty, and simulated Trust Fund revenues and expenditures are unlikely to be precise. For more information on our simulation methodology and the full range of results, see GAO-18-351.

Figure 2. Black Lung Disability Trust Fund Simulated Revenue and Black Lung Benefit Payments and Administrative Costs Based on Moderate Case Assumptions, Fiscal Years 2018 through 2050.

[23] This includes eliminating all cash assistance and medical benefits.

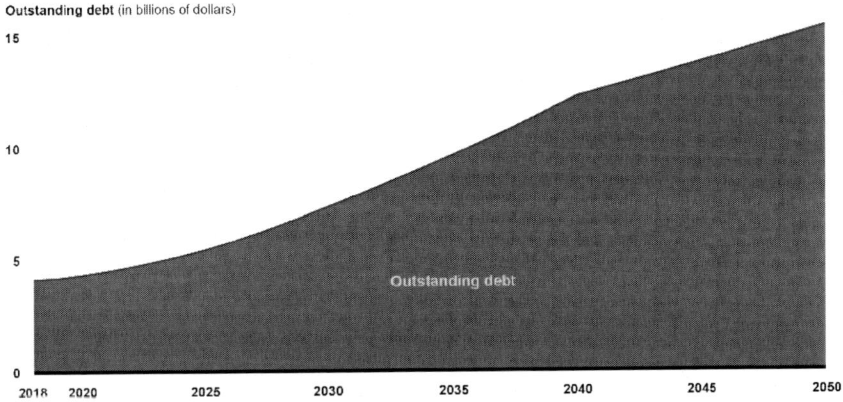

Source: GAO simulation based on data from the Department of Labor and Treasury, the Energy information Administration, and the Office of Management and Budget. | GAO-19-622T.

Notes: The principal amount of the Trust Fund's outstanding debt includes the principal amount of the Trust Fund's legacy debt—which was refinanced following the Energy Improvement and Extension Act of 2008 with repayment to be complete by fiscal year 2040—and the Trust Fund's annual borrowing from Treasury's general fund through 2050, which is simulated from fiscal years 2018 through 2050 and presented in nominal dollars. Moderate case simulations assumed that future coal production is consistent with the Energy Information Administration's reference case, which generally assumes trend improvement in known technologies, a view of economic and demographic trends that reflects the current central views of economic forecasters and demographers, and that current laws and regulations affecting the energy sector are unchanged through 2050. Moderate case simulations also assumed that future numbers of new black lung beneficiaries evolve over time based on the average growth rate for the period from fiscal years 2003 to 2015. Given the complexities of estimating future coal production and prices and new black lung beneficiaries, our simulations are subject to considerable uncertainty and simulated annual borrowing is unlikely to be precise. For more information on our simulations methodology and the full range of results, see GAO-18-351.

Figure 3. Black Lung Disability Trust Fund Simulated Principal Amount of Outstanding Debt to Treasury's General Fund Based on Moderate Case Assumptions, Fiscal Years 2018 through 2050.

Eliminating black lung benefits, however, would generally mean that coal tax revenue would be collected solely to fund the repayment of Trust Fund debt. As we reported in 2018, other options such as adjusting the coal tax and forgiving interest or debt, could also reduce future borrowing and improve the Trust Fund's financial position (see GAO-18-351).

Preliminary Observations Raise Concerns About DOL's Oversight of Coal Mine Operator Insurance

Federal law generally requires that coal operators secure their black lung benefit liability. Operators can purchase commercial insurance for this purpose or may self-insure if they meet certain DOL conditions. For example, self-insurers must obtain collateral in the form of an indemnity bond, deposit or trust, or letter of credit in an amount deemed necessary and sufficient by DOL to secure their liability.[24]

DOL officials said that the collateral they required from the five self-insured operators that filed for bankruptcy between 2014 and 2016 was inadequate to cover their benefit liabilities. For example, the collateral DOL required from Alpha Natural Resources was about 6 percent of its estimated benefit liability. As a result, approximately $185 million of estimated benefit liability was transferred to the Trust Fund, according to DOL data. We reviewed DOL documentation related to the five operator bankruptcies.[25] Table 1 shows the bankrupt operators; the amount of collateral each operator had at the time of bankruptcy; estimated benefit liability at the time of bankruptcy; and estimated benefit liability and number of beneficiaries that transferred to the Trust Fund, if applicable. Overall, three of these bankruptcies affected the Trust Fund, and two did not according to DOL. DOL officials told us that the bankruptcies of Arch Coal and Peabody Energy did not affect the Trust Fund because their benefit liabilities were assumed by the reorganized companies after emerging from bankruptcy.

---

[24] A letter of credit may only be used in conjunction with another acceptable form of collateral.

[25] We did not conduct a legal analysis of the relevant bankruptcy court dockets. Instead, we relied on documentation provided by DOL to describe these bankruptcies. DOL officials said that these were the self-insured operator bankruptcies that occurred from 2014 through 2016 that had the potential to affect the Trust Fund most in terms of total benefit liabilities that could be transferred to the Trust Fund, depending on the outcome of bankruptcy proceedings. DOL officials also included Walter Energy, but we excluded this company from our review because at the time of our review its bankruptcy proceeding had not progressed enough for us to assess the potential effect on the Trust Fund.

Table 1. Self-Insured Coal Operator Bankruptcies Reviewed, Filed from 2014 through 2016

Coal operator	Collateral at time of bankruptcy	Black lung benefit liability at time of bankruptcy	Estimated transfer of liability to Trust Fund	Estimated number of beneficiaries transferred to the Trust Fund
Alpha Natural Resources	$12 million	$206.6 million	$184.7 million	685
Arch Coal	$6.9 million	$90 million	$0	0
James River Coal Company	$0.4 million	$63.7 million to $75.9 million[a]	$62.8.million to $75 million	212
Patriot Coal	$15 million	$80 million	$65.1 million	687
Peabody Energy	$20 million	$68.4 million	$0	0

Source: DOL data, as confirmed by DOL officials. | GAO-19-622T.

Notes: In addition to collateral, DOL also in some cases received other funds, such as through a settlement agreement. Therefore, DOL's estimated loss to the Trust Fund may not equal estimated black lung benefit liability minus collateral. Estimates of operator liability and Trust Fund losses are based on projected payments over ensuing decades on existing and future claims, according to DOL officials.

[a] DOL and operator actuaries disputed James River Coal Company's estimated benefit liabilities and therefore DOL developed an estimated range of liability instead of an exact estimate.

As of June 2019, there are 22 operators that are self-insured and actively mining coal, according to DOL officials.[26] To ensure that the collateral they required from these operators was adequate to protect the Trust Fund, DOL officials said that they periodically reauthorized them which entailed, among other things, reviewing their most recent audited financial statements and claims information. DOL officials said that they prepared memos documenting these reviews and communicated with coal operators about whether their financial circumstances warranted increasing or decreasing their collateral. Table 2 provides information on the 22 self-insured operators including the date of each operator's most recent DOL reauthorization; the amount of DOL required collateral; and the operator's most recent estimated black lung benefit liability. Should any of these operators file for bankruptcy, they could also affect the Trust Fund because

[26] These include parent operators only. Subsidiaries of these operators may also be covered.

the amount of an operators' benefit liability that is not covered by collateral could also become the responsibility of the Trust Fund.

Table 2. Self-Insured Operator Reauthorization Date, Collateral, and Estimated Benefit Liability

Self-insured coal operator (from most recently reviewed by the Department of Labor (DOL), to least recently reviewed)	Date of most recent reauthorization	Collateral required by DOL to self-insure, as of September 2018	Most recent estimated black lung benefit liability
Coal operator 1	2018	$3.6 million	$18.4 million, as of 12/31/2017
Coal operator 2	2015	$1.1 million	No estimate available
Coal operator 3	2015	$2.5 million	$206 million, as of 8/03/2015
Coal operator 4	2014	$29.5 million	$109 million, as of 12/31/2016
Coal operator 5	2013	$8 million	No estimate available
Coal operator 6	2013	$1 million	No estimate available
Coal operator 7	2012	$8.4 million	$668,000, as of 1/1/1992
Coal operator 8	2012	$20.3 million	$68.4 million, as of 4/13/2016
Coal operator 9	2012	$1 million	No estimate available
Coal operator 10	2012	$15 million	No estimate available
Coal operator 11	2012	$21 million	$21.8 million, as of 12/31/2014
Coal operator 12	2011	$5.5 million	$47 million, as of 12/31/1984
Coal operator 13	2003	$0.4 million	No estimate available
Coal operator 14	2001	$0.8 million	$7.8 million, as of 01/01/1993
Coal operator 15	2000	$0.4 million	No estimate available
Coal operator 16	2000	$1.5 million	No estimate available[a]
Coal operator 17	1999	$1.4 million	No estimate available
Coal operator 18	1999	$29.2 million	No estimate available
Coal operator 19	1998	$6.9 million	$90 million, as of 12/31/2015
Coal operator 20	1997	$1.4 million	No estimate available
Coal operator 21	1994	$7.7 million	No estimate available
Coal operator 22	1988	$24.8 million	$15.1 million, as of 1/31/2005

Source: DOL data. | GAO-19-622T.

[a] According to DOL officials, this operator was acquired by another self-insured operator who assumed their benefit liability.

Preliminary analysis from our ongoing work indicates that DOL did not regularly monitor self-insured operators. Agency regulations state that DOL may adjust the amount of collateral required from self-insured operators when experience or changed conditions warrant. We reviewed

DOL's most recent reauthorization memos for each of the 22 operators. While some of these operators had been reauthorized more recently, we found that others had not been reauthorized by DOL in decades. One operator in particular had not been reauthorized by DOL since 1988. Additionally, for most of these operators, DOL either did not have estimates of their benefit liabilities, or the estimates were out of date (see table 2).

Beginning in summer 2015, DOL officials said that they stopped permitting any new coal mine operators to self-insure as the agency worked with auditors, economists, and actuaries to develop new procedures for self-insurance. At the same time, DOL generally stopped reauthorizing the 22 self-insured operators.[27] Earlier this year, two of these operators have filed for bankruptcy—Westmoreland Coal Company and Cloud Peak Energy—according to DOL officials. Additionally, due to deteriorating financial conditions, DOL recommended revoking another operator's self-insurance authority (Murray Energy).[28] However, Murray appealed this decision and DOL postponed responding to the appeal until their new self-insurance procedures are implemented, according to DOL officials.

DOL's new self-insurance procedures are currently being reviewed by OMB, and DOL officials said they did not know when they would likely be implemented. Until such procedures are implemented, DOL cannot ensure that the collateral it has required from self-insured operators is adequate to protect the Trust Fund should these operators become insolvent.

Chairwoman Adams, Ranking Member Byrne, and Members of the Subcommittee, this concludes my prepared statement. I would be happy to respond to any questions you may have at this time.

---

[27] DOL officials said that they reauthorized one of the 22 self-insured operators in 2018 to allow it to self-insure the legacy benefit liabilities of another operator that it had purchased.

[28] DOL regulations state that the agency, with good cause shown, may revoke the authorization of any self-insurer.

In: Key Government Reports. Volume 26 ISBN: 978-1-53616-568-5
Editor: Ernest Clark

Chapter 2

DOD HEALTH CARE: IMPROVEMENTS NEEDED FOR TRACKING COORDINATION OF SPECIALTY CARE REFERRALS FOR TRICARE PRIME BENEFICIARIES*

United States Government Accountability Office

ABBREVIATIONS

CLR	clear and legible report
DHA	Defense Health Agency
DOD	Department of Defense
NDAA 2017	National Defense Authorization Act for Fiscal Year 2017
MHS	Military Health System
MTF	military treatment facility
RMS	Referral Management Suite

* This is an edited, reformatted and augmented accessible version of the United States Government Accountability Office Report Report to Congressional Committees, Publication No. GAO-19-488, dated June 2019.

WHY GAO DID THIS STUDY

Specialty care referrals are a key component of care coordination for TRICARE Prime beneficiaries. Each Prime beneficiary is assigned to a primary care manager either at an MTF or within the civilian provider network. Primary care managers are responsible for overseeing all aspects of their patients' care, which includes making referrals for specialty care when needed.

The National Defense Authorization Act for Fiscal Year 2017 included a provision for GAO to examine care coordination within and between the direct and purchased care systems. Among other objectives, this chapter examines the extent to which the referral management process facilitates the coordination of primary and specialty care for TRICARE Prime beneficiaries. GAO examined relevant policies; analyzed current referral data from five MTFs it visited, selected for variety in military service, geographic location, and numbers of referrals; and interviewed officials with DHA and the military services. GAO also discussed the implementation of MHS Genesis with officials at DOD and the four MTFs where it has been implemented.

WHAT GAO RECOMMENDS

GAO recommends that the Secretary of Defense ensure that (1) MTF referral staff are trained to process and accurately document information in MHS Genesis about specially care referrals and (2) MHS Genesis is configured to produce reports with reliable data on the referral process. DOD concurred with both of these recommendations.

WHAT GAO FOUND

The Department of Defense's (DOD) Defense Health Agency (DHA) has limited information about the extent to which the referral management process facilitates the coordination of primary and specialty care for beneficiaries enrolled in TRICARE Prime—a managed care option—because information about their specialty care referrals is not always complete or accurate. The coordination of care for these beneficiaries is important because they may move between military treatment facilities (MTF) and civilian providers to obtain needed care. DHA requires specialty care providers to share documentation about the care they provided for referring primary care managers to review. This and other information is to be documented in the Referral Management Suite (RMS), the information technology system used by MTF officials to track and process referrals. However, GAO found that the five MTFs it visited had incomplete and unreliable data in RMS due to lack of training and insufficient staff. For example, GAO found that some MTFs were not tracking referral results in RMS due, in part, to lack of training. Officials with each of the military services told GAO that they are aware of RMS reliability issues and have been working to address them through system updates, training, and hiring staff.

DHA has begun to replace RMS and other existing information technology systems with Military Health System (MHS) Genesis, a new electronic health record system. The implementation of MHS Genesis began in 2017 at four MTFs, which have experienced difficulties with system implementation, including with referral management.

GAO found that the four MTFs using MHS Genesis were not adequately trained on how to use its referral management component prior to the system's deployment. This limited the MTFs' ability to process and track referrals, and led to concerns about the reliability of the system's referral data. While MHS Genesis training on referral management has been redesigned for the next round of MTFs slated for implementation in summer 2019, officials said that it remains unclear whether this training will provide the guidance needed for MTF officials to accurately process and capture information on specialty care referrals.

Without adequate training, DHA cannot ensure that the referral data in MHS Genesis accurately reflects the referral experiences of its Prime beneficiaries, potentially impacting the timeliness and quality of care they receive.

DHA and military service officials who are responsible for developing standardized referral management guidance for the department—the Referral Management Working Group—said that they have not been able to obtain reports about referrals for the four MTFs that use MHS Genesis. The system would need to be configured to produce the types of referral reports needed, according to these officials, who told GAO they have been working with the DHA officials responsible for system implementation to develop such reports. Without reliable reports on referrals, DHA will continue to lack the information it needs about the coordination of care for its TRICARE Prime beneficiaries, impeding its ability to manage referrals, as well as ensuring these beneficiaries receive needed care.

June 12, 2019

The Honorable James M. Inhofe
Chairman

The Honorable Jack Reed
Ranking Member
Committee on Armed Services
United States Senate

The Honorable Adam Smith
Chairman

The Honorable Mac Thornberry
Ranking Member
Committee on Armed Services
House of Representatives

In fiscal year 2018, the Department of Defense (DOD) offered health care services to more than 9 million eligible beneficiaries in the United States and abroad through TRICARE, its regionally structured health care program.[1] Under TRICARE, the department contracts with private sector companies—referred to as managed care support contractors (contractors)—to develop and maintain civilian provider networks and provide other services, such as specialty care referrals and claims processing.[2] Eligible beneficiaries can obtain primary and specialty health care services through the department's direct care system of military hospitals and clinics, referred to as military treatment facilities (MTF), or through its purchased care system of civilian providers.

Beneficiaries enrolled in TRICARE Prime, DOD's managed care option, must generally obtain referrals for their specialty care.[3] Referral management is a key component of care coordination for these beneficiaries because they may move between the direct and purchased care systems to obtain the care they need. TRICARE Prime beneficiaries are assigned to a primary care manager either at an MTF or within the civilian provider network. Primary care managers are responsible for overseeing all aspects of their patients' care, which includes making referrals for specialty care. To ensure the continuity of care for these beneficiaries, specialty care providers are required to share documentation about the care they provided during patients' visits for the referring primary care managers to review.[4]

---

[1] Eligible beneficiaries include active duty personnel and their dependents, medically eligible National Guard and Reserve servicemembers and their dependents, and retirees and their dependents and survivors. Active duty personnel include Reserve component members on active duty for at least 30 days.

[2] DOD has two TRICARE regions (East and West), and each region has its own contractor.

[3] Beginning on Jan. 1, 2018, TRICARE's non-Medicare-eligible beneficiary population could be enrolled in one of two basic health plan options—TRICARE Prime (a managed care option) or TRICARE Select (a self-managed, preferred provider option). This population includes all beneficiaries who do not meet the requirements for obtaining health care coverage under Medicare, which is generally available to people age 65 or older, younger people with disabilities, and people with end-stage renal disease.

[4] The process for submitting documentation of beneficiaries' care differs in the direct and purchased care systems. For example, MTF specialty care providers submit beneficiary information through the MTF's referral management center, which is responsible for processing and tracking all referrals.

As of March 2019, 5.1 million beneficiaries—over half of the eligible population—were enrolled in TRICARE Prime.

DOD's Defense Health Agency (DHA) administers the TRICARE program, which includes overseeing the contracts and setting policy for both the direct and purchased care systems, among other responsibilities. DHA is currently in the process of making changes to its information technology systems and to its organizational responsibilities—both of which will impact referral management. Since 2008, MTFs have primarily used an information technology system, called the Referral Management Suite (RMS), to process and track their specialty care referrals, according to DHA officials. In 2017, DHA began implementing Military Health System (MHS) Genesis, a new system that is designed to standardize electronic health records throughout DOD, and which will replace existing systems, including RMS. The implementation of MHS Genesis began at four MTFs, each of which has reportedly experienced difficulties with the system.[5]

Additionally, the National Defense Authorization Act for Fiscal Year 2017 (NDAA 2017), as amended, transferred administrative and management responsibility for MTFs from the military services' (Army, Navy, and Air Force) medical commands to DHA, including responsibility for referral management.[6] On Oct. 1, 2018, DHA initiated an incremental process for assuming these responsibilities and plans to complete this process by Oct. 1, 2021.[7]

---

[5] DHA plans to continue implementation at four additional sites on the West Coast by the end of calendar year 2019. The implementation of MHS Genesis is scheduled to be complete for all MTFs by the end of 2024.

[6] Within the direct care system, most MTFs are under the direction and control of their respective military service medical commands, including the Army Medical Command, the Navy Bureau of Medicine and Surgery, and the Air Force Major Commands. The Department of the Navy delivers health care to the Marine Corps. Pub. L. No. 114-328, § 702(a)(1), 130 Stat. 2000, 2193 (2016), codified, as amended, at 10 U.S.C. § 1073c.

[7] The John S. McCain National Defense Authorization Act for Fiscal Year 2019 (NDAA 2019) extended the date for the transfer of the administration of the MTFs to the DHA to September 30, 2021. Pub. L. No. 115-232, § 711 (a)(1). 132 Stat. 1636, (2018).

The NDAA 2017 included a provision for GAO to examine several issues related to DOD's delivery of health care, such as the coordination of care within and between the direct and purchased care systems.[8] In this chapter, we examine to what extent

1. the referral management process facilitates the coordination of primary and specialty care between the direct and purchased care systems for TRICARE Prime beneficiaries; and
2. DHA monitors TRICARE Prime specialty care referrals for the direct and purchased care systems.

To determine the extent to which the referral management process facilitates the coordination of care between the direct and purchased care systems for TRICARE Prime beneficiaries, we conducted site visits to a non-generalizable sample of five MTFs and reviewed and analyzed available RMS data on their specialty care referrals. The five MTFs included three MTFs representing each of the military services and an enhanced multi-service market area with two MTFs—Raymond W. Bliss Army Health Center (Fort Huachuca, Arizona), Naval Medical Center-San Diego (San Diego, California), 78th Medical Group (Robins Air Force Base, Georgia), and Brooke Army Medical Center and 59th Medical Wing Wilford Hall Ambulatory Surgical Center (Joint Base, San Antonio, Texas).[9] These MTFs were selected based on geographic diversity and a range in the numbers of specialty care referrals from the direct to the purchased care system. For these five MTFs, we analyzed RMS data on the extent to which documentation of beneficiaries' visits were submitted by the civilian specialty care providers for the MTF primary care managers from February 2017 to February 2018.[10]

---

[8] Pub. L. No. 114-328, § 751, 130 Stat. 2000, 2244-2245 (2016).

[9] Enhanced multi-service markets are multiple MTFs within the same geographic location that are organized under a single market manager and a unified business performance plan. Enhanced multi-service markets include San Antonio, Texas and the National Capitol Area, among others.

[10] Per DHA guidance, MTFs must close a referral with or without documentation of the beneficiary's visit to the civilian provider network within 180 days of the referral's

We also analyzed the available RMS data, for the MTFs we visited, from the MTF specialty care providers for the civilian network primary care managers.[11]

Additionally, we reviewed RMS data, for the MTFs we visited, on MTF's closure of specialty care referrals made from the direct to the purchased care system from December 2017 through July 2018.[12] We reviewed relevant documentation about RMS and interviewed knowledgeable officials about the accuracy and completeness of the system's data, which is discussed further in the report. We also reviewed DHA's July 2018 guidance for standardizing appointments and specialty care referrals, and relevant sections of the TRICARE Operations Manual.[13] We interviewed DHA and military service officials who participate in the Referral Management Working Group, which produces the department's referral management guidance, about how they use specialty care referral data in RMS to track the coordination of primary and specialty care.[14] We also reviewed documentation and interviewed relevant DHA and Referral Management Working Group officials about the department's transition to the new electronic health record system, MHS Genesis, to determine how this new system may impact the referral management process. Furthermore, we interviewed officials at the four MTFs where MHS

---

issuance. Therefore, we requested data for a complete year (February 2017-February 2018) because the end date was around 180 days prior to the July 2018 date of our data request.

[11] Civilian specialty care providers can be within or outside of the contractor's provider network and primary care managers are always within the contractor's provider network. As a result, we use the terms "civilian network primary care manager" and "civilian specialty care provider" throughout this report. A network provider is an individual or institutional provider that has a contract with the TRICARE contractor to provide care to TRICARE eligible beneficiaries.

[12] At the time of our review, DOD's guidance only addressed the closure of referrals from the direct to the purchased care system. Therefore, we did not examine data on the closure of other referrals, such as those made between providers in the direct care system. Further, in requesting a report with data on closure of referrals in August 2018, DHA officials told us that they had changed the report's methodology, and prior to December 2017, some data on this report would not be reliable.

[13] Defense Health Agency, Standard Appointing Processes, Procedures, Hours of Operation, Productivity, Performance Measures and Appointment Types in Primary, Specialty, and Behavioral Health Care in Medical Treatment Facilities (MTFs). Interim Procedures Memorandum 18-001 (Washington, D.C.: July 2018).

[14] While specialty care referrals can be made between civilian providers in the purchased care system, DHA and the military services do not play a role in coordinating this care.

Genesis has been implemented, and we compared how the MTFs' staff were trained to process referrals in MHS Genesis to federal standards for internal control related to developing competent individuals.[15]

Finally, we interviewed an official that represents military beneficiaries about their concerns regarding the referral process.[16]

To determine the extent to which DHA monitors TRICARE Prime specialty care referrals for the direct and purchased care systems, we reviewed the methodology DHA developed for assessing MTFs' performance with referrals generated in the direct care system, as well as the two subsequent quarterly performance reports using this methodology (April 2018 and August 2018).[17] We also reviewed DHA's July 2018 guidance for standardizing appointments and specialty care referrals that describes the monitoring responsibilities of DHA leadership, and we interviewed DHA officials about the data they use to monitor referrals. For purchased care referrals, we reviewed relevant sections of the managed care support contracts to identify contractors' referral management requirements, as well as their required monthly reports on referrals for the East Region (January through July 2018) and the West Region (May 2018 through July 2018).[18] We reviewed relevant documentation and interviewed DHA's TRICARE Health Plan officials, who conduct contractor oversight, about contractors' referral management requirements, and DHA's oversight structure and activities.

---

[15] GAO, *Standards for Internal Control in the Federal Government,* GAO-14-704G (Washington, D.C.: September 2014). Internal control is a process effected by an entity's oversight body, management, and other personnel that provides reasonable assurance that the objectives of an entity will be achieved.

[16] The Military Coalition is a group comprised of 32 organizations representing more than 5.5 million members of the uniformed services, including active duty, reservists, retirees, veterans, and their survivors and families.

[17] DHA developed the methodology in response to legislative requirements to standardize its medical appointment process. At the time of our study, the quarterly performance reports issued in April and August 2018 were the only two reports DHA had issued using that methodology.

[18] The shortened time frame for the West region was due to referral issues that began at the start of health care delivery in January 2018. These issues resulted in a waiver of certain requirements to help ensure timely access to specialty care through April 2018.

We also interviewed relevant contractor officials for both TRICARE regions about DHA's oversight of contract requirements for specialty care referrals.

We conducted this performance audit from April 2018 to June 2019 in accordance with generally accepted government auditing standards. Those standards require that we plan and perform the audit to obtain sufficient, appropriate evidence to provide a reasonable basis for our findings and conclusions based on our audit objectives.

We believe that the evidence obtained provides a reasonable basis for our findings and conclusions based on our audit objectives.

BACKGROUND

Referral Management Working Group

DHA and the military services work together on issues related to specialty care referrals through the Referral Management Working Group, which was established in September 2013.[19] According to its charter, the working group provides a forum for evaluating the referral process and making department-wide recommendations to

- optimize referral management through improved coordination within the direct care system and between the direct and purchased care systems;
- develop policies, business rules, training and other guidance on the management of referrals;
- establish new initiatives, technology, system changes, and electronic workflows related to the management of referrals; and

[19] The working group includes members from each of the military services (Army, Navy, and Air Force) and DHA.

- establish department-wide performance measures, including data sources, definitions and reports related to the management of referrals.

Referral Management Guidance and Requirements

As part of DHA's efforts to standardize the medical appointment process, including referral management, the Referral Management Working Group developed standardized guidance for the direct care system in 2017 that all of the military services are required to follow. Updated in July 2018, this guidance supersedes existing military-service-specific referral management policies. It outlines how the MTFs 1) process referrals within the direct care system, 2) how they send referrals to the purchased care system, and 3) how they process referrals received from the purchased care system. The guidance also addresses how these processes are to be documented in both RMS and MHS Genesis.

Each MTF has a referral management center that is responsible for processing specialty care referrals for its facility. DHA's guidance outlines how the MTFs' referral management centers are to facilitate the sharing of documentation about TRICARE Prime beneficiaries' care

- *from MTF specialty care providers:* When a referral management center accepts a specialty care referral from a civilian network primary care manager, the center is required to submit documentation of the beneficiary's visit—called "referral results"—from the MTF specialty care provider back to the civilian network primary care manager, and to track this submission in RMS or MHS Genesis.
- *to MTF primary care managers:* When an MTF primary care manager sends a referral to a civilian specialty care provider, the referral management center must follow up on required documentation the civilian specialty care provider is to submit about the beneficiary's visit, called a clear and legible report

(CLR).[20] The receipt of the report is documented in RMS or MHS Genesis.[21]

Historically, the contractors were responsible for following up on civilian specialty care providers' submission of CLRs to the MTFs' referral management centers. However, ultimately in 2013, the responsibility for this function was transferred to the MTFs' referral management centers. In order to follow up on a CLR, MTF officials must follow several steps, including checking the contractors' claims database to determine if the referral was used and contacting the specialty care provider multiple times to request the CLR. MTFs were given additional funding to address this new responsibility, and many continue to hire staff to carry out this function, according to Referral Management Working Group officials. Under the most current TRICARE contracts, DHA is requiring the contractors to have a process in place to address civilian specialty care providers that do not submit CLRs as required.

Separately, the TRICARE Operations Manual outlines referral requirements that both MTFs and the contractors must follow. The requirements are similar to those in DHA's July 2018 guidance, but include additional information for the contractors. For example, the manual includes specific requirements contractors must follow to ensure that specialty care referrals from a civilian network primary care manager are first offered to the local MTF to determine whether that MTF has the capability and capacity to provide the care. This process is called the "right of first refusal."[22]

---

[20] CLRs are specialty care consultation and referral reports, histories and physicals, progress notes, notes on episodes of care, other beneficiary information (such as laboratory reports), and discharge summaries for beneficiaries referred by MTFs to civilian specialty care providers.

[21] The CLRs are to be uploaded into DOD's Health Artifact and Image Management Solutions system, which is DOD's general repository for loading medical documentation, including consultation, laboratory, and radiology results.

[22] According to the TRICARE Operations Manual, capability is the scope of services the provider is both capable of performing and willing to perform, and capacity is the amount of time or number of services a provider is able to perform. MTFs' provide information on capability and capacity in documentation provided to the contractor.

Process for Specialty Care Referrals Made by Civilian Network Primary Care Managers

The process for referrals made by civilian network primary care managers varies depending on whether the referring MTFs have the capability and capacity to provide the specialty care:

- If a civilian network primary care manager generates a referral for specialty care, the contractor is required to contact the local MTF for the "right of first refusal." If the MTF does not have the capability and capacity to provide the care, the TRICARE Prime beneficiary obtains his or her care from a civilian specialty care provider who must submit a record of the beneficiary's visit to the referring primary care manager. Each contractor specifies its own requirements for civilian specialty care providers to submit this information to civilian network primary care managers.

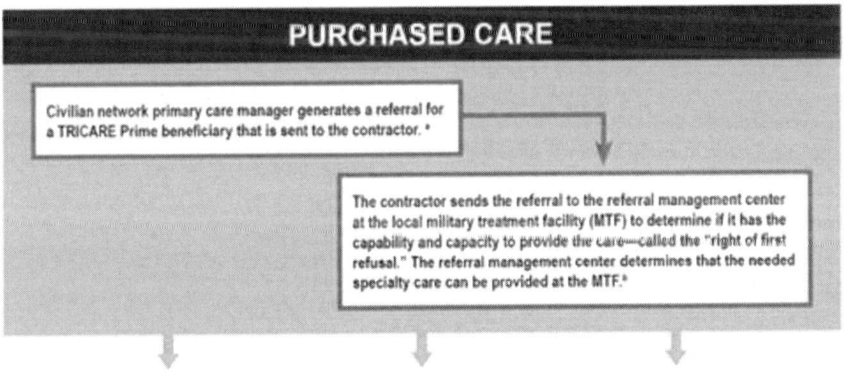

Figure 1. (Continued)

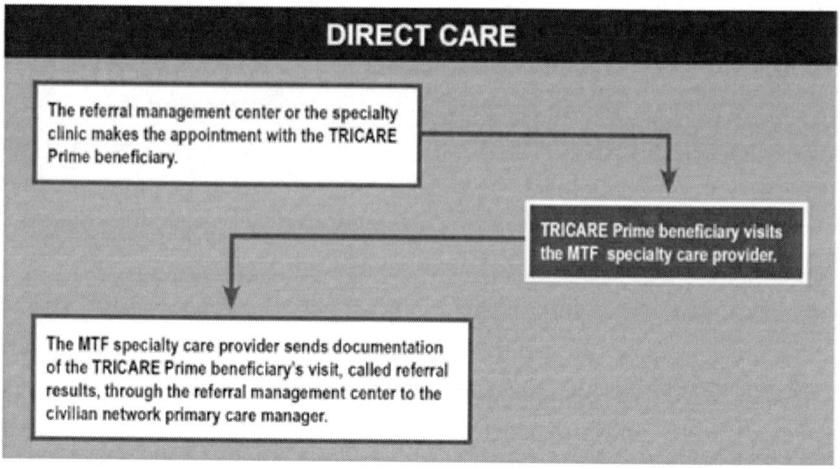

Source: GAO analysis of Department of Defense documents. | GAO-19-488.

Note: Direct care is the care received at military hospitals and clinics, referred to as MTFs, and purchased care is care received through a system of civilian provider networks. The Department of Defense (DOD) contracts with private sector companies—contractors— to develop and maintain civilian provider networks and provide other services, such as processing specialty care referrals. This figure represents the general process followed when a civilian network primary care manager makes a specialty care referral to the direct care system. However, these steps may change depending on several factors, such as whether the beneficiary lives near a military installation.

[a] Beneficiaries enrolled in TRICARE Prime, a managed care option, are assigned to a primary care manager either at an MTF or within the civilian provider network. Primary care managers are responsible for overseeing all aspects of their beneficiaries' care, which includes making referrals for specialty care when needed. Civilian primary care managers are within the contractor's provider network.

[b] Each MTF has a referral management center that is responsible for processing specialty care referrals for its facility. TRICARE defines capability as the scope of services the provider is both capable of performing and willing to perform, and capacity as the amount of time or number of services a provider is able to perform. As part of determining capacity, the referral management center must ensure that the specialty care appointment can be provided within TRICARE Prime's access-to-care standard of 28 days or less.

Figure 1. Process for Making a Specialty Care Referral for a TRICARE Prime Beneficiary from the Purchased to the Direct Care System.

- If a civilian network primary care manager generates a referral for specialty care that the MTF does have the capability and capacity to provide, the TRICARE Prime beneficiary may obtain his or her specialty care at the MTF.[23] After the beneficiary obtains care from the MTF specialty care provider, the MTF's referral management center is required to submit the referral results to the referring civilian network primary care manager. (See figure 1.)

Process for Specialty Care Referrals Made by MTF Primary Care Managers

Similarly, the process for referrals made by MTF primary care managers depends on whether the local MTF has the capability and capacity to provide the care:

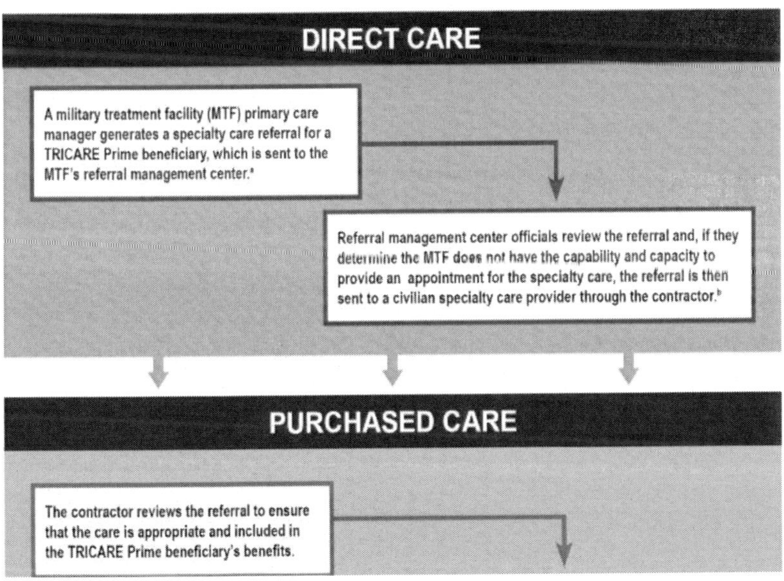

Figure 2. (Continued)

[23] The contractor consults current lists of MTF specialty care capabilities maintained by the MTF referral management center in order to facilitate the "right of first refusal" process.

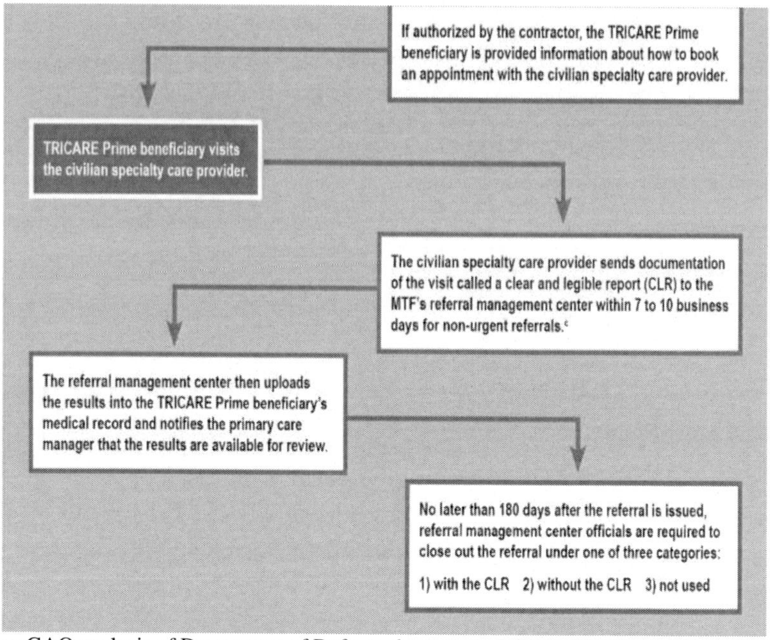

Source: GAO analysis of Department of Defense documents. I GAO-19-488.

Note: Direct care is the care received at military hospitals and clinics, referred to as MTFs, and purchased care is care received through a system of civilian provider networks. The Department of Defense (DOD) contracts with private sector companies—contractors— to develop and maintain civilian provider networks and provide other services, such as processing specialty care referrals. This figure represents the general process followed when an MTF primary care manager makes a specialty care referral to the purchased care system.

[a] Beneficiaries enrolled in TRICARE Prime, a managed care option, are assigned to a primary care manager either at an MTF or within the civilian provider network. Primary care managers are responsible for overseeing all aspects of their beneficiaries' care, which includes making referrals for specialty care when needed. Each MTF has a referral management center that is responsible for processing specialty care referrals for its facility.

[b] The TRICARE program defines capability as the scope of services the provider is both capable of performing and willing to perform, and capacity as the amount of time or number of services a provider is able to perform. As part of determining capacity, the referral management center must ensure that the specialty care appointment can be provided within TRICARE Prime's access to care standards of 28 days or less.

[c] CLRs are specialty care consultation and referral reports, histories and physicals, progress notes, notes on episodes of care, other beneficiary information (such as laboratory reports), and discharge summaries for beneficiaries referred by MTFs to civilian specialty care providers.

Figure 2. Process for Making a Specialty Care Referral for a TRICARE Prime Beneficiary from the Direct to the Purchased Care System.

- If a primary care manager at the MTF generates a referral for specialty care that the MTF has the capability and capacity to provide, the TRICARE Prime beneficiary obtains his or her care from the MTF specialty care provider. MTF specialty care providers are not required to submit documentation of the beneficiary's visit to the referring primary care manager because they share the same electronic health record system.
- If a primary care manager at the MTF generates a referral for specialty care that the MTF does not have the capability and capacity to provide, the TRICARE Prime beneficiary may obtain his or her care from a civilian specialty care provider, who must submit a CLR to the MTF for the primary care manager to review. Each contractor specifies the time frame in which the CLR must be provided.[24] The required time frame is the same for both TRICARE regions—2 days for urgent care referrals, and 7 to 10 days for all other referrals. (See figure 2)

MTFs' Requirements for Closing Referrals

MTFs' referral management centers are required to enter referral disposition information into RMS (or MHS Genesis, once implemented) to indicate whether the referral was used. According to DHA's guidance, referral management centers are responsible for closing referrals from their facilities to civilian specialty care providers within 180 days of the referrals' issuance. In contrast, MTFs currently are not explicitly required to close referrals made by their primary care manager to their specialty care providers or referrals generated by the "right of first refusal" process. However, DHA plans to include additional requirements for closing these referrals in its updated guidance, according to officials.[25]

---

24 Each contractor develops a provider handbook to outline the roles and responsibilities of civilian providers both within and outside of its network.

25 Officials from the Referral Management Working Group told us that they are currently developing an update to this guidance that should be completed by July 2019. Additionally, DOD is in the process of making changes to streamline its TRICARE Prime referral process

DHA Has Limited Information about the Extent to Which the Referral Process Facilitates the Coordination of Care between the Direct and Purchased Care Systems for TRICARE Prime Beneficiaries

Referral Data Was Incomplete and Unreliable for the MTFs Reviewed, and the Reports Examined Did Not Accurately Reflect the Referral Process

DHA has limited information about the extent to which the referral process facilitates the coordination of care for TRICARE Prime beneficiaries between the direct and purchased care system based on issues we identified with the completeness and reliability of the data and reports we reviewed from RMS. Specifically, we found that the five MTFs we visited had incomplete and unreliable data in RMS about receipt of CLRs, the submission of specialty care referral results, and the closure of specialty care referrals. In addition, we found that the RMS reports used by the Referral Management Working Group were not reliable for assessing certain aspects of the referral process due, in part, to unreliable data in RMS as well as a flawed methodology. The Referral Management Working Group, which includes officials from DHA and the military services' medical commands, acknowledged the limitations of this referral data in RMS. Officials with the military services' medical commands told us that they have been meeting routinely with their MTFs' referral management centers to help address issues with the reliability of RMS data.

---

in response to recent legislation. For example, the NDAA 2017 requires DOD to allow non-active duty TRICARE Prime beneficiaries to use urgent care facilities without the need for a specialty care preauthorization. In addition, the NDAA 2019 requires DOD to streamline the referral process for TRICARE Prime beneficiaries in calendar year 2019.

CLRs

We found that the CLR data in RMS for the five MTFs we visited were incomplete. As a result, the referral management center officials at these MTFs could not accurately determine if they received CLRs for all referrals they sent to civilian specialty care providers as required by DHA's guidance. For example, the RMS data we reviewed indicated that these MTFs received between 20 to 77 percent of the CLRs they expected.[26] Officials from one MTF told us that their CLR data in RMS was incomplete because the MTF did not have enough staff to follow up on CLRs that had not been received, which they described as a time-intensive process. These officials told us that they recently hired contract staff to begin the process of following up on CLRs for specialty care referrals. In addition, the RMS data for another MTF indicated that they had received less than half of their CLRs (45 percent), but officials from this MTF told us they thought they had received almost all of their CLRs and could not explain the difference.

Specialty Care Referral Results

We found that the submission of specialty care referral results was generally not being tracked in RMS, as required by DHA's guidance for the three MTFs we visited that accept these referrals.[27] As a result, information in RMS about the submission of referral results is incomplete, limiting MTFs' ability to determine whether MTFs have been submitting all specialty care referral results as required. Officials from the three MTFs told us that although they submitted their referral results, they generally had not been using RMS to track the submission of this information. Instead, officials with two of the MTFs told us that they used the contractors' database to track referral results because RMS has had ongoing issues with receiving required data from its administrative system, which is used for scheduling

---

[26] Our analysis of CLRs received did not include referrals that had not been used.

[27] Two of the five MTFs we visited are small facilities and do not accept purchased-todirect care referrals because they do not have the capability.

appointments, among other things.[28] However, officials from the two MTFs told us that these issues have been resolved as of January 2019, and since that time they had begun using RMS to track referral results. Further, officials with the remaining MTF told us that they previously tracked this information in a spreadsheet, but they recently learned how to track it in RMS. According to a Referral Management Working Group official, RMS is capable of tracking the submission of specialty care referral results, but MTF officials may not understand how to use this capability.

Closure of Specialty Care Referrals

We found that RMS data on the closure of specialty care referrals (from MTF primary care managers to civilian specialty care providers) for the five MTFs we visited was unreliable due to inconsistencies we identified between the RMS data we reviewed and MTF officials' statements about the closed referrals for their facility. As a result, these MTFs may have difficulty determining whether their referrals had been used and whether they closed these referrals within 180 days as required by DHA guidance. For example, one MTF had closed around 75 percent of its referrals in RMS as "not used." However, officials at this MTF told us that many of these referrals were likely used, but were closed as "not used" because staff needed to close referrals in RMS quickly and did not have time to determine the referrals' status. Officials we spoke with at another MTF told us they did not understand the full capabilities of RMS and had not been using this data to determine whether or not they had closed their specialty care referrals. A third MTF told us they closed all of its referrals within the required time frame of 180 days; however, we found that only about half of its referrals were documented as closed in RMS. Officials at this MTF could not explain this discrepancy.[29]

---

[28] The Composite Health Care System allows clinicians to electronically perform patient appointment processes and scheduling, order laboratory tests, authorize radiology procedures, and prescribe medications.

[29] In April 2019, an official from this MTF told us that the MTF has fixed this discrepancy in RMS, although officials still could not explain why it occurred.

RMS Reports

In 2017, the Referral Management Working Group began monitoring MTFs' RMS data as part of its effort to develop DHA's initial standardized guidance for appointments and referral management. Officials with the Referral Management Working Group told us that two reports from RMS—the CLR Percent Received Report and the Referral Performance Report—have been used to assess the receipt of CLRs and closure of specialty care referrals.[30] For the MTFs we visited, we found the CLR Percent Received Report to be unreliable in determining whether CLRs were received due to both the report's flawed methodology and MTFs' input of inaccurate information into RMS.[31] Officials with the working group acknowledged the limitations of this chapter and told us that they supplement this information with another RMS report, the Referral Performance Report, which they use to review the closure of specialty care referrals. However, when we reviewed the CLR and specialty care referral closure data in the Referral Performance Report, we also identified inaccuracies with these data.[32] For example, we found that several MTFs had closed more direct-to-purchased care referrals than they had issued. Officials with the Referral Management Working Group explained that some MTFs are inaccurately inputting data into RMS. As a result, there are inaccuracies in the Referral Performance Reports, such as referrals that are double counted. Officials said that these MTFs will need to be trained on how to accurately input data into RMS.

Officials with each of the military services' medical commands who participate in the Referral Management Working Group told us that they began taking steps to address their concerns about the reliability of RMS data in an effort to implement the standardized appointment and referral

---

[30] DHA officials who maintain information technology systems develop the methodology for these reports in consultation with the Referral Management Working Group, according to working group officials.

[31] The methodology for the CLR Percent Received report removes referrals from the denominator when the referrals have been closed as either "not used" or "without a CLR." Therefore, the results on the number CLRs received may be artificially inflated because the number of referrals without a CLR are removed from the overall calculation.

[32] The Referral Performance Reports have more than 40 data elements. We reviewed the six elements in the report that related to the closure of direct-to-purchased care referrals and obtaining CLRs.

guidance at their MTFs. They have worked with DHA on two updates to RMS—one in March 2018 and one in January 2019—in an effort to address some of these data concerns.[33] In addition, they have been reviewing and discussing data with their MTFs' referral management center officials, sometimes through their regional officials, on a monthly or quarterly basis to discuss available RMS data, including data on CLRs and closures of referrals, among other things. Further, the military service medical commands are working to help their MTFs obtain more staff to pursue outstanding CLRs. In addition, the medical commands are focused on teaching their MTFs' referral management center staff to correctly input referrals and avoid inadvertent double counting.

Inadequate Training on Processing Referrals in MHS Genesis Has Contributed to Data Reliability Concerns for Four Pilot MTFs; Updates to the System Are Planned

DHA's initial implementation of MHS Genesis—which will replace RMS and other systems—did not include adequate training for referral management, resulting in concerns about data reliability. Specifically, referral management center officials with the four MTFs using MHS Genesis told us that although training was provided on the use of the system, this training did not adequately address the use of the system's referral management component prior to its deployment. These officials told us they generally trained themselves and most developed their own training materials on the system, which requires a different referral processing workflow than RMS. This lack of training limited MTFs' ability to use MHS Genesis to evaluate their performance and led to MTF officials' concerns about the reliability of the system's referral data. For example, officials at two of the MTFs told us that their staff had not been provided training on how to aggregate data on the receipt of CLRs even though MHS Genesis is capable of generating this chapter. As a result,

[33] These updates included improved transmission of data from the Composite Health Care System and updates to beneficiary categories.

their staff manually tracked the receipt of individual CLRs, not only increasing the risk of errors, but also making it more difficult to assess their facilities' overall performance. An MTF official at one of these facilities told us that the CLR report from MHS Genesis was likely unreliable because staff had not received formal training on how to accurately use the system to input and process referral data. Federal standards for internal control highlight the importance of training to develop staff competencies appropriate for key roles.[34] Without adequate training, DHA cannot ensure that the data and reports derived from MHS Genesis accurately reflect the referral experiences of its TRICARE Prime beneficiaries, or whether any remediation is needed with regard to the process.

MTF officials also told us that it took longer to process referrals in MHS Genesis, and as a result, some MTFs had to add staff to their referral management centers or extend the centers' hours to process referrals within required time frames. The Referral Management Working Group told us that they are working with DHA officials to upgrade the referral management component of the MHS Genesis system to help improve the referral process. A DHA official responsible for system implementation stated that standardized training will be developed and provided to MTF staff to correspond with the upgrade, which the official anticipates will be implemented in summer 2020. In the interim, this official told us that they have redesigned the MHS Genesis training on referral management, which DHA plans to use for the MTFs included in the next wave of MHS Genesis implementation in summer 2019. However, Referral Management Working Group officials are unclear whether the redesigned training will address the concerns expressed by the MTFs currently using the system.

Furthermore, Referral Management Working Group officials told us that they have not been able to obtain reports about referrals for MTFs that use MHS Genesis. Working group officials explained that MHS Genesis may be capable of producing the types of referral reports they need, but the system would need to be configured by DHA to do so. These officials told

---

[34] GAO-14-704G.

us that they have been working with the DHA officials who are overseeing system implementation to identify the data and methodology needed to develop reports on specialty care referrals, including information on CLRs, referral results, and specialty care referral closures. Working group officials said that they were aware that MHS Genesis already produces a report on CLRs received, but they were concerned about using it because they had been cautioned by MTF officials that the report contained inaccurate data. As an initial step, these officials told us that they requested the methodology for this chapter in order to determine its accuracy; however, as of March 2019, they had not received this information. Federal standards for internal control state that management should use quality information to achieve its objectives. Quality information is obtained through relevant data from reliable sources in a timely manner based on the identified information requirements.[35] Without reliable reports on specialty care referrals, the Referral Management Working Group may have difficulties not only determining TRICARE Prime beneficiaries' use of referrals, but also fulfilling its goals of optimizing and standardizing the referral management process.

DHA's Monitoring of TRICARE Prime Specialty Care Referrals in the Direct Care System Is Expected to Evolve and in the Purchased Care System Is Focused on Contractors' Reports

DHA's Monitoring of TRICARE Prime Specialty Care Referrals for the Direct Care System Is Limited, but Expected to Evolve as DHA Assumes Administrative Responsibilities for MTFs

DHA, through its Clinical Business Operations branch, monitors TRICARE Prime specialty care referrals for the direct care system.

[35] GAO-14-704G.

Specifically, DHA uses one of the 15 metrics it established based on its requirement to standardize appointments across MTFs—the average number of days elapsed from referral to appointment booked.[36] This metric is derived from the MHS Dashboard, which contains MTF health care performance measures based on data from DHA's current electronic health record system.[37] DHA plans to monitor a second metric related to referrals—average days from referral to appointment decision or send to a civilian specialty care provider—when they obtain additional staff. DHA's current approach for monitoring direct care system referrals is expected to evolve as it assumes administrative responsibilities for the remaining MTFs, but DHA has not yet determined its new organizational structure or its corresponding staffing needs. DHA's July 2018 standardized appointment and referral management guidance assigned oversight responsibilities for referrals to Regional Commands, which would be a new organizational structure within DHA. However, according to a DHA official, the Regional Command structure is no longer being considered, and DHA is now pursuing a different organizational structure that is in the process of being approved. As a result, DHA has not determined the staffing it would need, including the staff needed to monitor specialty care referrals for TRICARE Prime beneficiaries. In addition, DHA has not yet determined the monitoring activities that would be conducted by its staff versus the military services, according to DHA officials.

DHA Uses Required Monthly Reports from Its Contractors to Oversee Referrals in Its Purchased Care System

Within DHA's TRICARE Health Plan Division, referral management officials monitor contractors' performance on purchased care referrals by

---

[36] Other measures include the percent of demand for care that was unmet within a given month and the percentage of appointments that were leaked to the network, which occurs when the MTF has the capability to provide specialty care, such as orthopedics but sends the referral to a civilian specialty care provider.

[37] Data posted to the MHS Dashboard is extracted from the MHS Data Repository. The MHS Dashboard does not contain data for the four MTFs at which MHS Genesis has been deployed.

reviewing data in three required referral management reports the contractors submit on a monthly basis. These reports include:

1. the "preauthorization/authorization and referral timeliness/ accuracy" report that provides information on the total number of referrals that met timeliness and accuracy requirements in the previous month;
2. the "right of first refusal" report that indicates the number of referrals accepted and declined by each MTF via this process in the previous month; and
3. the "directed referrals" report that provides information on care provided by network and non-network specialty care providers in a geographic area where a specific specialty may not be available from a network specialty care provider.

When any of the reports demonstrate that a contractor is not meeting its requirements, DHA officials said that they may ask the contractor to implement a corrective action plan. For example, at the January 2018 start of health care delivery to TRICARE beneficiaries in the West region, DHA officials found that the contractor's performance on referral processing timeliness failed to meet contract requirements and was inadequate to meet the overall demand for specialty care referrals. According to DHA officials, the contractor was managing about 8,000 referrals a day, and within a few weeks, the contractor had a queue of 70,000 referrals that needed to be processed. DHA officials instituted a corrective action requiring the contractor to submit daily referral processing status reports in addition to their monthly reports. They also instituted a waiver that allowed TRICARE Prime beneficiaries to see a civilian specialty care provider without an authorized referral from the contractor. The waiver was removed in April 2018 based on information in the contractor's daily reports, which indicated that the contractor had eliminated the backlog and was meeting referral processing timeliness requirements.

As DHA's organizational structure evolves, it plans to modify its organizational responsibilities for monitoring contractors' performance.

DHA's TRICARE Health Plan Division has been using a regional structure—the TRICARE Regional Offices (East and West)—to conduct oversight of contractors' performance in meeting certain contract requirements, including those for referrals. However, in 2018, DHA began the process of collapsing oversight responsibilities across the regions.[38] As a result, certain regional officials now oversee their specific area of responsibility, such as specialty care referrals, for the entire U.S. and do not focus solely on their individual region.

CONCLUSION

The referral management process is a key component of care coordination for TRICARE Prime beneficiaries who may move between the direct and purchased care systems to obtain needed specialty care. However, our review of selected MTFs' referral data revealed that DHA does not know the extent to which care is being coordinated for this population because MTFs' referral management centers do not always document accurate and complete referral information in RMS due to a lack of staff and the need for additional training. Furthermore, some of the RMS reports used by the Referral Management Working Group are based on data that are not reliable and a methodology that does not accurately reflect key information. Consequently, military service officials with the Referral Management Working Group have been working with DHA and their MTFs to improve the reliability of RMS data through system updates, training, and hiring staff.

It will also be important for DHA to ensure that the types of problems experienced with RMS do not recur with MHS Genesis. However, the four MTFs using MHS Genesis have already experienced difficulties with processing and tracking referral information due, at least in part, to the lack

[38] DHA's TRICARE Health Plan office is organized into several components, each of which is responsible for distinct areas of contractor oversight for a distinct region (East and West). As part of its reorganization in 2018, DHA began moving away from a regional division of responsibility for its staff. While some components have implemented this change, as of March 2019, not all components have done so.

of adequate training. While MHS Genesis training on referral management has been redesigned for the next round of MTFs slated for implementation in summer 2019, it remains unclear whether this training will provide the guidance needed for MTF officials to accurately process and capture information on specialty care referrals. Without adequate training on processing referrals in MHS Genesis, DHA increases its risk that the data and reports derived from the system may not accurately reflect the referral experiences of its TRICARE Prime beneficiaries.

As DHA assumes administrative responsibilities for all MTFs, developing reports for MHS Genesis that accurately reflect TRICARE Prime beneficiaries' referral experiences will become even more paramount. Without this, the Referral Management Working Group will continue to be hampered in its ability to update DHA's referral management guidance that is intended to standardize the referral management process across all MTFs. Further, DHA will continue to lack accurate information it needs to determine whether the referral management process is facilitating the delivery of timely and quality care to its TRICARE Prime beneficiary population through effective care coordination.

Recommendation for Executive Action

- The Secretary of Defense should direct DHA to ensure that MTFs' referral management center staff are trained to process and accurately document information in MHS Genesis about specialty care referrals, including the receipt of CLRs, the submission of referral results, and the closure of referrals. (Recommendation 1)
- The Secretary of Defense should direct DHA to ensure that MHS Genesis is configured to produce reports that accurately reflect the use and outcomes of specialty care referrals. (Recommendation 2)

AGENCY COMMENTS

DOD provided written comments on a draft of this chapter, which are reprinted in appendix I. DOD also provided technical comments, which we incorporated as appropriate. In its written comments, DOD concurred with both of our recommendations and noted that DHA has worked with the MHS Genesis program office to improve training and reporting. DOD stated that DHA will assess the effectiveness of the improved training when MHS Genesis is rolled out to the next wave of MTFs starting in fiscal year 2020 and will make additional training and reporting improvements as subsequent waves of MTFs are transitioned to MHS Genesis through fiscal year 2024.

We are sending copies of this chapter to the Acting Secretary of Defense and appropriate congressional committees.

Debra A. Draper
Director, Health Care

APPENDIX I: COMMENTS FROM THE DEPARTMENT OF DEFENSE

OFFICE OF THE ASSISTANT SECRETARY OF DEFENSE

1200 DEFENSE PENTAGON
WASHINGTON, DC 20301-1200

HEALTH AFFAIRS

MAY 2 3 2019

Ms. Debra Draper
Director, Health Care
U. S. Government Accountability Office
441 G St., NW
Washington, DC 20548

Dear Ms. Draper:

This is the Department of Defense (DoD) response to the Government Accountability Office (GAO) Draft Report, GAO-19-488, "DOD HEALTH CARE: Improvements Needed for Tracking Coordination of Specialty Care Referrals for TRICARE Prime Beneficiaries" dated April 29, 2019 (GAO Code 102752).

Thank you for the opportunity to provide management comments (attached) on the draft report recommendations. We appreciate the in-depth review and findings related to the processes for monitoring the care coordination of specialty care referrals. The DoD concurs with both of the GAO recommendations focused on ensuring military Medical Treatment Facility referral staff are trained to process and accurately document specialty care information in Military Health System (MHS) GENESIS and that MHS GENESIS is configured to produce reports with reliable data on the referral process. The Defense Health Agency has worked with the MHS GENESIS program office to improve training and reporting and will assess the effectiveness of the improved training in the Wave 1 MHS GENESIS roll-out starting in Fiscal Year (FY) 2020 and will make additional training and reporting improvements in subsequent waves through FY 2024.

We sincerely thank the GAO team members for developing this report and for the steadfast commitment to protecting the health and wellness of our Service members, civilian workforce, and beneficiaries.

Sincerely,

Tom McCaffery
Principal Deputy Assistant Secretary of Defense (Health Affairs)

In: Key Government Reports. Volume 26 ISBN: 978-1-53616-568-5
Editor: Ernest Clark

Chapter 3

VA HEALTH CARE: ESTIMATING RESOURCES NEEDED TO PROVIDE COMMUNITY CARE*

United States Government Accountability Office

ABBREVIATIONS

CHAMPVA	Civilian Health and Medical Program of the Department of Veterans Affairs
EHCPM	Enrollee Health Care Projection Model
OMB	Office of Management and Budget
VA	Department of Veterans Affairs
VHA	Veterans Health Administration

* This is an edited, reformatted and augmented version of United States Government Accountability Office; Report to Congressional Requesters; Accessible Version, Publication No. GAO-19-478, dated June 2019.

Why GAO Did This Study

VA continues to focus on the use of community care to address challenges with veterans' access to health care services at VA medical facilities. In fiscal year 2019, VA plans to consolidate the Veterans Choice Program and several other community care programs under a single new Veterans Community Care Program. GAO and others have previously reported on past challenges VA has faced regarding the reliability, transparency, and consistency of its budget estimates for health care.

GAO was asked to review VA's use of community care and efforts to develop budget estimates for this care. This chapter describes (1) trends in obligations for and utilization of VA's community care programs since fiscal year 2014, (2) how VA develops its community care budget estimate and any subsequent changes made to this estimate, and (3) how VA's actual obligations for community care compared with estimated obligations for fiscal years 2017 and 2018.

GAO reviewed actual obligation and utilization data for fiscal years 2014 through 2018, as well as estimated obligations for fiscal years 2019 through 2021. GAO also reviewed available VA documentation on the methods and data used to develop VA's community care budget estimate that informed the President's budget request for fiscal years 2017 through 2019. GAO also interviewed VA officials and contractors responsible for developing these estimates, and OMB staff responsible for the federal budget.

VA and OMB reviewed a draft of this chapter. VA's technical comments were incorporated as appropriate.

What GAO Found

To help ensure that veterans are provided timely and accessible health care services, the Department of Veterans Affairs (VA) may purchase care from non- VA providers, known as community care. VA obligated $14.9

billion for community care in fiscal year 2018, an increase of $6.7 billion (about 82 percent) since fiscal year 2014. The number of veterans authorized to use community care increased from 1.3 million to 1.8 million during this period. By fiscal year 2021, VA estimated obligations to increase to $17.8 billion, and officials estimate at least 1.8 million veterans will continue to use this care.

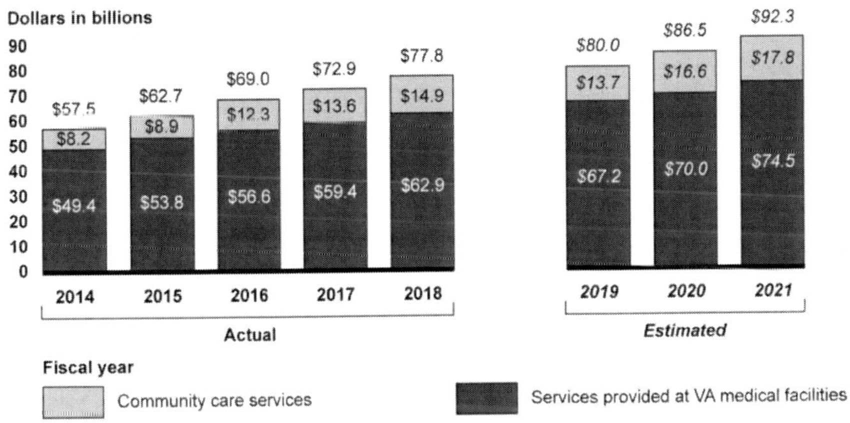

Source: GAO analysis of Department of Veterans Affairs (VA) data. | GAO-19-478.

Note: VA estimated obligations for fiscal year 2019 to reflect $1.8 billion in anticipated savings as a result of a VA policy change regarding the timing of certain community care obligations.

VA Health Care Obligations, Fiscal Years 2014 through 2021.

VA uses a projection model to estimate the majority of resources needed to provide health care services. Beginning with the President's fiscal year 2018 budget request, VA updated its model to estimate the resources needed to purchase over 40 community care services accounting for over 75 percent of VA's community care budget estimate. These services include outpatient and inpatient care, among others. For the remainder of its community care budget estimate, which includes nursing care in state-operated homes, VA uses other methods based on historical utilization. VA's budget estimate is successively reviewed at VA and the Office of Management and Budget (OMB) to inform the President's budget request. VA identified several changes made during the review process to its budget estimate for fiscal years 2018 and 2019 to reflect more current information related to utilization and costs, among other factors. VA's actual obligations for community care for fiscal years 2017 and 2018 were $1.2 billion and $2.2 billion higher, respectively, than originally estimated. According to VA officials, this occurred for several reasons, including policy changes and increased costs for the Veterans Choice Program. To support higher obligations, VA requested and received additional funding for the Veterans Choice Program outside the annual appropriations process and used other funding sources, such as unobligated amounts from prior fiscal years.

June 12, 2019

The Honorable Jon Tester
Ranking Member
Committee on Veterans' Affairs
United States Senate

The Honorable Mark Takano
Chairman

The Honorable Phil Roe
Ranking Member
Committee on Veterans' Affairs
House of Representative

The Department of Veterans Affairs (VA) operates one of the nation's largest health care delivery systems. In fiscal year 2018, VA provided care to over 6.9 million patients—mostly, veterans—and obligated about $78 billion for that care.[1] The majority of veterans utilizing VA health care services receive care in VA-operated medical facilities, including 170 VA

---

[1] Veterans account for around 6.2 million of the 6.9 million VA patients. Patients are individuals treated at a VA medical facility or whose treatment is paid for by VA. Patients include veterans and their beneficiaries; active duty military; reserve personnel; and VA employees.

medical centers and over 1,000 outpatient facilities. However, veterans may also obtain services from non-VA providers in the community—known as community care—through one of several community care programs aimed at helping ensure veterans receive timely and accessible care.[2]

In the last 5 years, Congress has taken steps to expand the availability of community care for veterans. The Veterans Access, Choice, and Accountability Act of 2014 created the temporary Veterans Choice Program (Choice Program) and provided $10 billion in funding for veterans to obtain health care services from community providers when veterans faced long wait times or travel distances, or had other challenges accessing care at VA medical facilities.[3] Implemented in fiscal year 2015, the temporary authority and funding of the Choice Program was separate from that of other previously existing programs through which VA has the option to purchase care from community providers.[4] In 2018, the VA MISSION Act was enacted requiring VA to implement within one year a permanent community care program—the Veterans Community Care Program—that consolidates the Choice Program along with several other community care programs.[5] The act, among other things, requires VA to ensure veterans can receive timely and accessible community care when certain criteria are met. The act also requires VA to issue regulations—including defining certain eligibility criteria—to carry out the Veterans Community Care Program.[6]

---

[2] For the purposes of this report, unless otherwise indicated, the terms "community care" and "community providers" refer, respectively, to the services the department purchases outside VA medical facilities for veterans and other eligible beneficiaries, and the non-VA providers who deliver the services. Other eligible beneficiaries include veterans' spouses and dependent children that receive care from community providers under certain VA health care programs. Additionally, for the purposes of this report, "community care programs" includes programs and activities that provide community care whether under statutory or under contractual authority.

[3] Pub. L. No. 113-146, §§ 101, 802, 128 Stat. 1754, 1755-1765, 1802-1803 (2014).

[4] VA implemented the Choice Program in November 2014.

[5] John S. McCain III, Daniel K. Akaka, and Samuel R. Johnson VA Maintaining Internal Systems and Strengthening Integrated Outside Networks Act of 2018. Pub. L.No. 115- 182, tit. I, 132 Stat. 1393 (2018) (VA MISSION Act).

[6] For example, in February 2019, VA proposed new access standards based on average drive times and wait times. For primary and mental health care services, VA is proposing a 30-minute average drive time standard and wait-time standard of 20 days. For specialty care,

The amount of funding VA receives for community care and other health care services is predominately determined as part of the annual appropriations process. In preparation, VA must annually develop an estimate of the resources needed to provide community care and other health care services for two fiscal years—known as its health care budget estimate.[7] This budget estimate is one step in a complex, multistep budget formulation process that culminates in an appropriations request for VA health care in the President's annual budget request to Congress. Developing this estimate is inherently complex, as assumptions and imperfect information are used to project the likely quantity and cost of the health care services VA expects to provide. These projections are made 3 and 4 years into the future using data from the most recently completed fiscal year. As such, VA's budget estimate is prepared in the context of uncertainties about the future—not only about program and veterans' needs, but also about future economic conditions, presidential policies, and congressional actions that may affect the funding needs in the year for which the request is made. As a result of these uncertainties, the amount of resources VA obligates during a fiscal year for health care services may be different than the amount it estimates it will obligate in its annual budget estimate.[8]

We and others have previously identified challenges VA has faced regarding the reliability, transparency, and consistency of its budget estimates for medical services used to support the President's budget request. For example, in February 2012, we reported that VA's estimated savings from operational improvements for providing medical services—used to support both the President's budget request for fiscal year 2012 and VA's advance appropriations request for fiscal year 2013—lacked

VA is proposing a 60-minute average drive time standard and wait-time standard of 28 days. 84 Fed. Reg. 5629 (Feb. 22, 2019).

[7] VA's annual appropriations for health care include advance appropriations that become available one fiscal year after the fiscal year for which the appropriations act was enacted.

[8] An obligation is "a definite commitment that creates a legal liability of the government for the payment of goods and services ordered or received, or a legal duty on the part of the United States that could mature into a legal liability by virtue of actions on the part of the other party beyond the control of the United States." See GAO, *A Glossary of Terms Used in the Federal Budget Process*, GAO-05-734SP (Washington, D.C.: Sept. 1, 2005).

analytical support or were flawed, raising questions regarding the reliability of the estimated savings.[9] Due to these issues and other concerns related to veterans receiving timely care, we concluded that VA health care is a high-risk area and added it to our High Risk List in 2015.[10]

In light of these challenges and as VA looks to implement the VA MISSION Act to consolidate a number of its community care programs for veterans into a single program, you asked us to review VA's use of community care, as well as its efforts to develop a budget estimate for this care. In this chapter, we describe

1) trends in obligations for and utilization of VA's community care programs since fiscal year 2014,
2) how VA develops its estimate of the resources needed for community care and any subsequent changes made to this estimate, and
3) how VA's actual obligations for community care compared to its estimated obligations for fiscal years 2017 and 2018.

To describe trends in obligations for VA's community care programs since fiscal year 2014, we reviewed data from VA's budget justifications and other data provided by VA on actual obligations for fiscal years 2014 through 2018—the most recently completed fiscal year for which these data were available.[11] We also reviewed the budget justification data on

---

[9] See GAO, *VA Health Care: Challenges in Budget Formulation and Execution*, GAO-09-459T (Washington, D.C.: March 12, 2009); *VA Health Care: Methodology for Estimating and Process for Tracking Savings Need Improvement*, GAO-12-305 (Washington, D.C.: Feb. 27, 2012); and *VA's Health Care Budget: In Response to a Projected Funding Gap in Fiscal Year 2015, VA Has Made Efforts to Better Manage Future Budgets*, GAO-16-584 (Washington, D.C.: June 3, 2016). See also VA Office of Inspector General, *Veterans Health Administration: Audit of Non-VA Medical Care Obligations* (Washington, D.C.: Jan. 12, 2016).

[10] GAO maintains a high-risk program to focus attention on government operations that it identifies as high risk due to their greater vulnerabilities to fraud, waste, abuse, and mismanagement or the need for transformation to address economy, efficiency, or effectiveness challenges. See GAO, *High-Risk Series: Substantial Efforts Needed to Achieve Greater Progress on High Risk Areas*, GAO-19-157SP (Washington, D.C.: March 6, 2019).

[11] The budget justification provides Congress with estimates and other information that support the policies and spending decisions represented in the President's budget request, including

estimated obligations for fiscal years 2019 through 2021.[12] The community care data we reviewed reflected obligations for all VA community care programs for veterans and other eligible beneficiaries, such as spouses and dependent children. For comparison purposes, we reviewed data on VA's total obligations for health care services, including care provided in VA medical facilities and community care. We also reviewed data on actual obligations by service type—such as dental care, inpatient care, long-term care, outpatient care, and prosthetics.[13] To describe trends in utilization of community care programs, we reviewed VA data on the number of veterans authorized to use community care services, and the types and number of community care services those veterans actually used from fiscal years 2014 through 2018.[14] We also reviewed data on the actual utilization of community care by other eligible beneficiaries from fiscal years 2014 through 2018.

To describe how VA develops its estimate of the resources needed for community care and any subsequent changes made to this estimate, we reviewed and analyzed the VA's budget justifications for the President's budget requests for fiscal years 2017 through 2019, which was the latest fiscal year for which complete information were available to support the President's budget request.[15] VA documents we reviewed included those that describe the methods and types of data used to develop VA's

---

information on what VA plans to achieve with the resources requested. In particular, VA's budget justification includes detailed information on estimates of funding needed for ongoing health care services and health-care-related initiatives proposed by the Secretary of Veterans Affairs and the President. As such, VA's budget justification is used to provide Congress with important information about agency priorities, as well as the implications of the requested amounts for VA's provision of health care services to veterans.

[12] Estimated obligations for fiscal year 2021 informed the advance appropriation request for that fiscal year.

[13] According to VA officials, the actual obligation amounts for certain service types for fiscal years 2016 through 2018 were understated due to the way certain adjustments were accounted for in VA's financial management system.

[14] Except for certain emergency and pharmacy care, all community care services for veterans must be authorized in advance of when veterans access the care in order for claims to be paid. Data we reviewed on veterans represents the number of individuals who had at least one authorization to receive community care during the fiscal year. Each authorization may result in multiple appointments, and a single veteran may have multiple authorizations under different community care programs.

[15] The President's budget request for fiscal year 2020 and advance appropriation for 2021 was released on March 11, 2019.

community care budget estimates. VA data we reviewed included the community care budget estimates projected by those methodologies and changes made to those estimates that informed the President's budget request.

To describe how VA's actual obligations for community care compared to its estimated obligations for fiscal years 2017 and 2018, we reviewed data from VA's budget justifications and other data provided by VA on estimated and actual obligations for community care for those years. We chose this period because 2017 was the first fiscal year estimates of obligations for community care were reported separately in VA's budget justifications, and 2018 was the most recently completed fiscal year for which data were available. The community care data we reviewed reflected obligations for all VA community care programs for veterans and other eligible beneficiaries, including data by service type.

For all objectives, we spoke with officials from the Veterans Health Administration's (VHA) Office of Finance, Office of Community Care, and the Office of Enrollment and Forecasting within the Office of the Assistant Deputy Under Secretary for Health for Policy & Planning; VA's actuarial consultant for developing health care budget estimates; and the Office of Management and Budget (OMB). Additionally, we assessed the reliability of the VA data, including data on obligations for and utilization of health care services, by checking for missing values and outliers, and interviewed relevant VA officials who are knowledgeable about these data. As a result of these steps, we determined that the data were sufficiently reliable for the purpose of our reporting objectives.

We conducted this performance audit from April 2018 through June 2019 in accordance with generally accepted government auditing standards.

Those standards require that we plan and perform our work to obtain sufficient, appropriate evidence to provide a reasonable basis for our findings and conclusions based on our audit objectives. We believe that the evidence obtained provides a reasonable basis for our findings and conclusions based on our audit objectives.

Background

VA's Community Care Programs and Planned Consolidation

VA has purchased health care services from community providers since as early as 1945. In general, veterans may be eligible for community care when they are faced with long wait times or travel long distances for appointments at VA medical facilities, or when a VA medical facility is unable to provide certain specialty care services, such as cardiology or orthopedics. In general, community care services must be authorized in advance of when veterans access the care.[16]

Currently, there are several community care programs through which VA purchases hospital care and medical services for veterans, including the Choice Program. In implementing the VA MISSION Act, VA plans to consolidate four of its community care programs for veterans under the Veterans Community Care Program, which is expected to go into effect by June 2019. (See Table 1.)

VA also provides health care services to veterans and other eligible beneficiaries through community providers under additional benefit programs. These benefit programs include the Civilian Health and Medical Program of the Department of Veterans Affairs (CHAMPVA) and the Camp Lejeune Family Member Program, among others.[17] After implementing the VA MISSION Act, VA will continue to operate the community care programs for other eligible beneficiaries, such as

---

[16] Except for certain emergency and pharmacy care, all community care services for veterans must be authorized in advance of when veterans access the care in order for claims to be paid. Among other things, the authorization informs the community provider of the veteran's medical needs and the specific services that will be covered, as well as the period of validity (i.e., beginning and ending dates) for the episode of care. Each authorization may result in multiple appointments, and a single veteran may have multiple authorizations under different community care programs.

[17] CHAMPVA is a comprehensive health care program that provides health care coverage for spouses and children of veterans who were permanently and totally disabled, or died, from a service-connected disability, or of those veterans who died in the line of duty. Camp Lejeune Family Member Program provides reimbursement to family members of certain veterans for health care costs associated with specific medical conditions.

CHAMPVA and others, as it has historically done. Appendix I contains more information about VA's community care programs.

Table 1. Description of four Department of Veterans Affairs community care programs expected to be consolidated under the Veterans Community Care Program, beginning June 2019

VA Community Care Program	Program description
Dialysis contracts	In June 2013, VA awarded contracts to numerous community providers nationwide to deliver dialysis—a life-saving medical procedure for patients with end stage renal disease (permanent kidney failure). When dialysis services are not feasibly available at VA medical facilities, veterans may be referred to one of VA's contracted dialysis providers, and veterans may receive dialysis at local clinics on an outpatient basis, or at home (if the contractors offer home-based dialysis services).
Individually authorized care	Started in 1945, the program is the primary means by which VA has traditionally purchased community care.[a] Local VA medical center staff determine veteran eligibility, create authorizations, and assist veterans in arranging care with community providers that are willing to accept VA payment.
Patient-Centered Community Care	Created in 2013 under existing statutory authority and fully implemented in April 2014. VA awarded contracts to two, third-party administrators in September 2013 to develop regional networks of community providers to deliver specialty care, mental health care, limited emergency care, and maternity and limited newborn care when such care is not feasibly available from a VA medical facility.
Veterans Choice Program	Created by the Veterans Access, Choice, and Accountability Act of 2014, introduced in November 2014, and expanded in April 2015 and December 2015.[b] VA modified its contracts with the two Patient-Centered Community Care third-party administrators to establish networks of community providers, schedule appointments with community providers for veterans, and pay community providers for their services.

Source: GAO analysis of Department of Veterans Affairs (VA) information. | GAO-19-478.

Note: In this table, "community care programs" includes programs and activities that provide community care whether under statutory or under contractual authority.

[a]38 U.S.C. § 1703.

[b]Pub. L. No. 113-146, 128 Stat. 1754 (2014).

Developing a Budget Estimate for VA Health Care

The amount of funding VA receives to provide its health care services is determined during the annual appropriations process. In preparation for the process, VA develops an estimate of the resources needed to provide its health care services—known as its health care budget estimate—for two fiscal years.[18] This budget estimate is one step in a complex, multistep budget formulation process, which culminates in an appropriation request for VA health care that updates the earlier, advance appropriation request for the upcoming fiscal year and an advance appropriation request for the next fiscal year in the President's annual budget request to Congress.

VA's health care budget estimate includes the total cost of providing health care services, including direct patient costs, as well as costs associated with management, administration, and maintenance of facilities. VA uses its Enrollee Health Care Projection Model (EHCPM) to estimate the majority of resources needed to meet the expected demand for health care services, and uses other methods for the remaining services.[19] VA uses the EHCPM to make projections 3 and 4 years into the future for budget purposes based on data from the most recent fiscal year. For example, in 2017, VA used data from fiscal year 2016 to develop its health care budget estimate for the fiscal year 2019 request and advance appropriation request for fiscal year 2020.[20] The EHCPM's estimates are based on three basic components: (1) the projected number of veterans who will be enrolled in VA health care, (2) the projected quantity of health care services enrollees are expected to use, and (3) the projected unit cost of providing these services.[21] Each component is subject to a number of complex adjustments

---

[18] VA's annual appropriations for health care include advance appropriations that become available one fiscal year after the fiscal year for which the appropriations act was enacted.

[19] The EHCPM was developed in 1998 by VA and its actuarial consultant. For the fiscal year 2019 request, the EHCPM estimated resources for 79 health care services available in VA medical facilities or through community care, which accounted for nearly 95 percent of VA's total health care budget estimate.

[20] Similarly, VA used data from fiscal year 2015 to develop its health care budget estimate for the fiscal year 2018 request and advance appropriation request for fiscal year 2019.

[21] Unit costs are the costs to VA of providing a unit of service, such as a 30-day supply of a prescription or a day of care at a medical facility.

to account for the characteristics of VA health care and the veterans who access VA's health care services. (See Figure 1.)

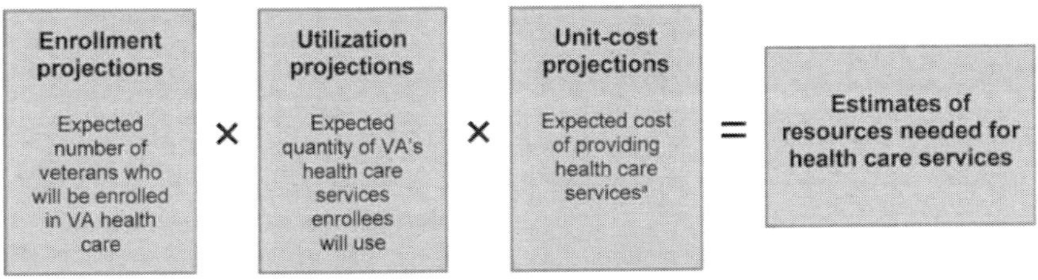

Source: GAO analysis of Department of Veterans Affairs (VA) information. | GAO-19-478.

Notes: The EHCPM makes a number of complex adjustments to projections for VA's health care services to account for the characteristics of VA health care and enrolled veterans. For example, the EHCPM includes adjustments to account for reliance on VA health care, that is, the extent to which enrolled veterans will choose to access health care services through VA as opposed to other health care programs or insurers. Additionally, the EHCPM includes adjustments to incorporate the age, gender, priority level, and geographic location of enrolled veterans.

[a]VA calculates the cost of providing a unit of service in different ways depending on the type of service provided. For example, unit costs for some pharmacy services reflect the cost of a 30-day supply of a prescription, and unit costs for inpatient services reflect the cost of a day of care at an inpatient facility.

Figure 1. Basic Components of VA's Enrollee Health Care Projection Model (EHCPM).

VA uses other methods to estimate resources needed for the remaining portion of its budget estimate. This portion of the budget includes the state home per diem program, CHAMPVA, and other health care programs for veterans and other eligible beneficiaries, as well as health- care-related initiatives proposed by the Secretary of Veterans Affairs or the President.[22] (See app. II for more information about the other methods VA uses in developing its health care budget estimate.)

[22] Under the state home per diem program, veterans may receive nursing home, domiciliary, or adult day care in state veterans homes. These facilities are owned and operated by state governments. Each state establishes eligibility and admission criteria for its homes and VA provides payment on a per diem basis for eligible veterans.

Table 2. Review process resulting in the President's budget request for the Department of Veterans Affairs

Date	Budget formulation event
Year one	
April-September	VA's Office of Budget issues guidance, on behalf of the Secretary of Veterans Affairs, for preparing a budget submission.
	The Veterans Health Administration (VHA) develops most of its health care budget estimate using the Enrollee Health Care Projection Model based on data from the most recently completed fiscal year. VHA develops the remainder of its health care budget estimate using other methods.
	VHA uses the budget estimate to inform its budget submission for health care, which is subsequently reviewed by the VHA Undersecretary for Health.
	The Secretary reviews and approves the budget submission for health care along with the submissions from other components of VA.
September	VA delivers the budget submission to the Office of Management and Budget (OMB).
October-December	OMB reviews VA's budget submission and issues a decision on funding and policy priorities for VA. VA may appeal this decision.
Year two	
January	OMB prepares the President's budget request, and VA concurrently prepares its budget justification, which supports the policies and funding decisions in the President's budget request.
Early February	The President submits the budget request, which includes requested resources for VA health care, to Congress.
October 1	The fiscal year begins.

Source: GAO analysis and presentation of Department of Veterans Affairs (VA) and OMB information | GAO-19-478.

Note: VHA administers VA's health care system. VHA is one of three administrations that comprise VA and are included in the President's budget request for VA: VHA, the Veterans Benefits Administration, and the National Cemetery Administration.

VHA generally starts to develop a health care budget estimate approximately 10 months before the President submits the budget to Congress, which should occur no later than the first Monday in February.[23] The budget estimate changes during the 10-month budget formulation process, in part, due to successively higher levels of review in VA and

[23] 31 U.S.C. § 1105(a). VHA administers VA's health care system. VHA is one of three administrations that comprise VA and are included in the President's budget request for VA: VHA, the Veterans Benefits Administration, and the National Cemetery Administration.

OMB before the President's budget request is submitted to Congress. (See Table 2.) The Secretary of Veterans Affairs considers the health care budget estimate developed by VHA when assessing resource requirements among competing interests within VA, and OMB considers overall resource needs and competing priorities of other agencies when deciding the level of funding requested for VA's health care services.

OMB passes back decisions, known as a "passback," to VA and other agencies on their budget estimate, along with funding and policy proposals to be included in the President's budget request. VA has an opportunity to appeal the passback decisions before OMB finalizes the President's budget request. Concurrently, VA prepares a congressional budget justification that provides details supporting the policy and funding decisions in the President's budget request.

As of fiscal year 2017, VA primarily receives funding for all health care it provides or purchases through the following appropriation accounts:

- Medical Services: health care services provided to eligible veterans and other beneficiaries in VA facilities and non-VA facilities, among other things.
- Medical Community Care: health care services that VA authorizes for veterans and other beneficiaries to receive from community providers.[24]
- Medical Support and Compliance: the administration of the medical, hospital, nursing home, domiciliary, supply, and research activities authorized under VA's health care system, among other things.
- Medical Facilities: the operation and maintenance of VHA's capital infrastructure, such as the costs associated with nonrecurring maintenance, leases, utilities, facility repair, laundry services, and groundskeeping, among other things.[25]

---

[24] The VA Budget and Choice Improvement Act required the inclusion of an appropriation account specifically for community care starting with the President's fiscal year 2017 budget request. Pub. L. No. 114-41, tit. IV, § 4003, 129 Stat. 443, 462-463 (2015).

[25] Nonrecurring maintenance is designed to correct, replace, upgrade, and modernize existing infrastructure and utility systems.

Separate from VA's health care appropriation accounts, the Veterans Access, Choice, and Accountability Act of 2014 provided $10 billion in funding for the Choice Program, which was implemented in early fiscal year 2015 and authorized until funds were exhausted or through August 7, 2017, whichever occurred first.[26] However, VA received additional authority and funding to maintain the Choice Program through June 6, 2019, when the new Veterans Community Care Program is expected to go into effect.[27] VA expects that the new Veterans Community Care Program will be primarily funded through the Medical Community Care appropriation account.

VA OBLIGATIONS FOR AND NUMBER OF VETERANS AUTHORIZED TO USE COMMUNITY CARE HAVE GROWN FROM FISCAL YEAR 2014 THROUGH FISCAL YEAR 2018

VA's Obligations for Community Care Increased by Over 80 Percent from Fiscal Years 2014 through 2018, and VA Estimates Obligations Will Grow an Additional 20 Percent through 2021

Our analysis of VA budget justification data shows that from fiscal year 2014 through fiscal year 2018, the total amount VA actually obligated

---

[26] Pub. L. No. 113-146, §§ 101(p), 802, 128 Stat. 1754, 1755-1765, 1802-1803 (2014).

[27] Additional funding for the Choice Program was provided on three separate occasions. Legislation enacted in August and December of 2017 provided an additional $4.2 billion for the Veterans Choice Fund. VA Choice and Quality Employment Act of 2017, Pub. L. No. 115-46, § 101, 131 Stat. 958, 959 (2017) (providing an additional $2.1 billion for the Veterans Choice Fund); An Act to amend the Homeland Security Act of 2002 to require the Secretary of Homeland Security to issue Department of Homeland Security-wide guidance and develop training programs as part of the Department of Homeland Security Blue Campaign, and for other purposes, Pub. L. No. 115-96. Div. D, § 4001, 131 Stat. 2044, 2052-53 (2017) (providing an additional $2.1 billion for the Veterans Choice Fund). In addition, the VA MISSION Act provided an additional $5.2 billion for the Veterans Choice Fund and authorized VA, beginning March 1, 2019, to use remaining amounts in the Fund for the Community Care Program, along with any other available amounts in other appropriation accounts for such purposes. Pub. L. No. 115-182, §§142, 510, 132 Stat. 1393, ** (2018).

for community care increased 82 percent, from $8.2 billion to $14.9 billion.[28] Since VA implemented the Choice Program in fiscal year 2015, the share of VA's obligations for community care relative to VA's total obligations for health care services increased through fiscal year 2018, from about 14 to 19 percent of VA's total obligations for health care services. By fiscal year 2021, VA estimates that the total amount obligated for community care will increase to $17.8 billion, an increase of about 20 percent from the $14.9 billion in actual obligations for fiscal year 2018.[29] (See Figure 2).

As Figure 2 shows, the largest increase in actual obligations for community care occurred from fiscal years 2015 through 2016, when they increased by $3.4 billion, from $8.9 billion to $12.3 billion. According to VA officials, this increase in obligations during this period reflected veterans' expanded use of community care through the Choice Program, as more providers participated in the provider networks established by third-party administrators or entered into provider agreements with VA facilities.[30] (Figure 3 provides information on VA's obligations for community care by the Choice Program and by other community care programs.) The increase in actual obligations for community care from fiscal year 2016 through fiscal year 2017 was also largely due to expanded use of community care through the Choice Program.

---

[28] For fiscal years 2014, 2015, and 2016, we examined data for community care obligations for the Veterans Choice Fund and the Medical Services Appropriation account. For fiscal years 2017 and 2018, we examined data for community care obligations for the Veterans Choice Fund and the Medical Community Care appropriation account.

[29] For fiscal year 2019, we examined data for community care obligations for the Veterans Choice Fund and the Medical Community Care appropriation account. For fiscal years 2020 and 2021, we examined data for community care obligations for the Medical Community Care appropriation account.

[30] Provider agreements are agreements with community providers to provide health care services to veterans eligible under the Veterans Choice Program. VA establishes provider agreements, schedules veterans' appointments, and reimburses the providers directly (using Choice Program funds) when the third party administrators fail to schedule veterans' appointments within the time frames required by VA policy. See GAO, *Veterans' Choice Program: Improvements Needed to Address Access-Related Challenges as VA Plans Consolidation of its Community Care Programs,* GAO-18-281 (Washington, D.C.: June 4, 2018).

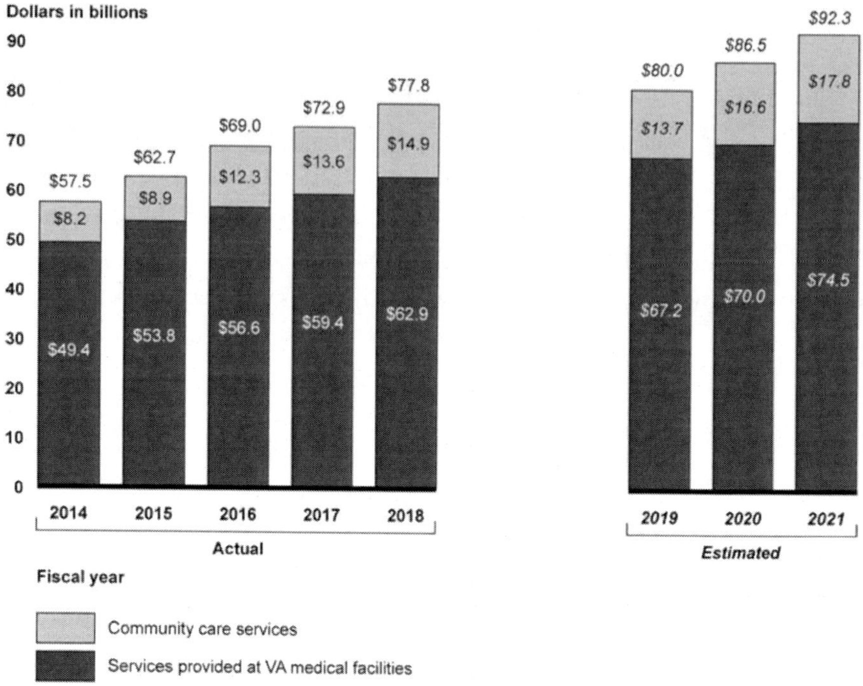

Source: GAO analysis of Department of Veterans Affairs (VA) data. | GAO-19-478.

Notes: Numbers may not sum to totals due to rounding. Community care services refer to the services that VA purchases outside VA medical facilities for veterans and other eligible beneficiaries. Data reflect actual obligations from fiscal years 2014 through 2018, and estimated obligations from fiscal years 2019 through 2021. VA estimated obligations for fiscal year 2019 to reflect $1.8 billion in anticipated savings as a result of a VA policy change regarding the timing of certain community care obligations.

Figure 2. Department of Veterans Affairs' Obligations for Community Care as a Share of Total Obligations for VA Health Care Services, Fiscal Years 2014 through 2021.

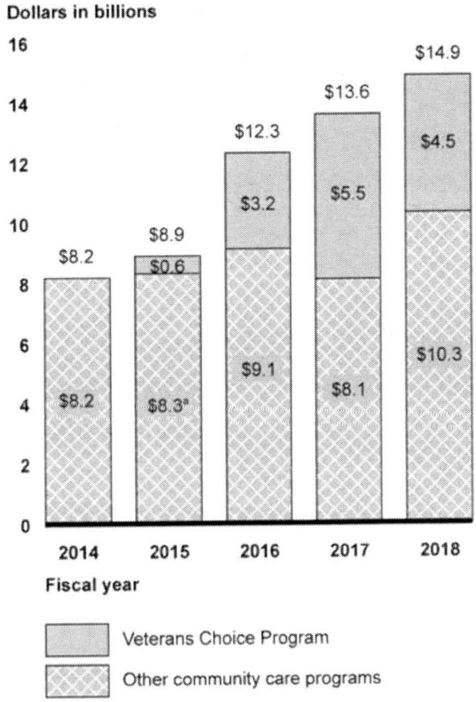

Source: GAO analysis of Department of Veterans Affairs (VA) data. | GAO-19-478.

Notes: Amounts may not add up due to rounding. The Veterans Choice Program that was established to provide care in the community for veterans began in fiscal year 2015. "Other community care programs" include the Civilian Health and Medical Program of the Department of Veterans Affairs and other benefit programs under which VA provides care for veterans and other eligible beneficiaries, such as spouses and dependent children, through community providers. VA estimates that obligations for community care will total $13.7 billion in fiscal year 2019, which reflects $1.8 billion of anticipated savings as a result of a VA policy change regarding the timing of certain community care obligations.

[a]This amount includes $739 million in Veterans Choice Program funds obligated by VA between May 1, 2015, and September 30, 2015, for other VA community care programs. Congress granted VA authority to use Veteran Choice Program funds for this purpose in July 2015. See Pub. L. No. 114-41, § 4004(a), 129 Stat. 443, 463 (2015).

Figure 3. Department of Veterans Affairs' Actual Community Care Obligations for the Veterans Choice Program and Other Community Care Programs, Fiscal Years 2014 through 2018.

VA officials attributed this increase to efforts to obligate as much of the available Choice Program funding as possible before the anticipated end of the Choice Program in August of 2017. From fiscal years 2017 through 2018, obligations for community care continued to increase, but the increase was partially due to greater use of other community care programs, according to VA officials.

From fiscal years 2014 through 2018, the increases in total actual obligations for VA community care were driven largely by increases in obligations for outpatient and inpatient services.[31] Over this time period, VA's actual obligations for outpatient services increased by $2 billion, from $2.3 billion to $4.3 billion, and actual obligations for inpatient services increased by $818 million, from $1.8 billion to $2.7 billion.[32] Figure 4 illustrates how outpatient and inpatient services accounted for most of VA's total community care obligations for fiscal year 2018.

VA estimated that from fiscal years 2019 through 2021, obligations for community care will increase to $17.8 billion, which VA officials said are attributable to the new eligibility criteria under the VA MISSION Act.[33] The authority for the Choice Program ends June 6, 2019, after which the new Veterans Community Care Program—which consolidates VA's community care programs under the VA MISSION Act—will be expected to begin. For comparison purposes, the largest increase in obligations for services provided at VA medical facilities is estimated to occur between fiscal years 2020 and 2021. VA officials said this increase is attributable, in part, to efforts related to hiring and telehealth in response to the eligibility criteria under the VA MISSION Act.

---

[31] Outpatient services include services such as immunizations and vision exams, and inpatient services include services such as surgeries.

[32] According to VA officials, the actual obligation amounts for certain service types for fiscal years 2016 through 2018 were understated due to the way certain adjustments were accounted for in VA's financial management system. These adjustments were $1.2 billion for fiscal year 2016; $700 million for fiscal year 2017; and $2.2 billion for fiscal year 2018.

[33] For example, in February 2019, VA proposed new access standards based on average drive times and wait times. For primary care, mental health, and non-institutional extended care services, VA is proposing a 30-minute average drive time standard and wait-time standard of 20 days. For specialty care, VA is proposing a 60-minute average drive time standard and wait-time standard of 28 days.

The Number of Veterans Authorized to Use Community Care Increased about 40 Percent from Fiscal Years 2014 through 2018

Our analysis of VA data on authorizations for community care shows that the number of veterans authorized to use community care increased 41 percent from fiscal years 2014 through 2018.[34] (See Figure 5.) The approximately 1.8 million veterans authorized to use community care in 2018 represented about 30 percent of all veterans accessing VA health care services that year (approximately 6.2 million veterans).[35] By fiscal year 2021, VA officials told us that they estimate that at least 1.8 million veterans will still use community care.[36]

Our analysis of VA data also shows that after being authorized for care, veterans' utilization of certain community care services increased from fiscal years 2014 through 2018. Over this time period, a number of outpatient services experienced increases of more than 200 percent in utilization, especially chiropractic visits (418 percent, from 143,000 to 743,000 visits), physical therapy visits (252 percent, from 857,000 to 3 million visits), and non-mental health related office visits (243 percent, from 651,000 to 2.2 million visits). In comparison, our analysis found relatively smaller increases in veteran utilization for certain inpatient services. For example, the utilization for surgical inpatient stays increased about 39 percent—from 253,000 to 352,000 bed days.

---

34 Data we reviewed on veterans represents the number of individuals who had at least one authorization to receive community care during the fiscal year. Among other things, the authorization informs the community provider of the veteran's medical needs and the specific services that will be covered, as well as the period of validity (i.e., beginning and ending dates) for the episode of care. Each authorization may result in multiple appointments, and a single veteran may have multiple authorizations under different community care programs.

35 In addition to veterans, we found that the number of other eligible beneficiaries, such as spouses and dependents, that used community care increased from 342,000 to 404,000— an 18 percent increase—from fiscal years 2014 through 2018. Data we reviewed on other eligible beneficiaries represents the number of individuals who received community care through one of the benefits programs during the fiscal year.

36 VA officials said this estimate does not account for the new eligibility criteria under the VA MISSION Act.

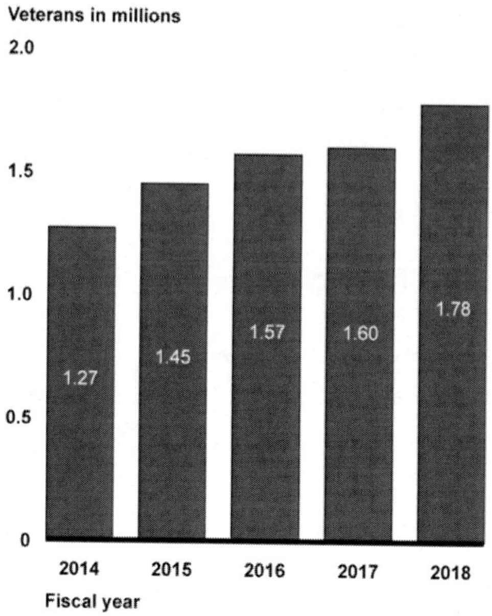

Source: GAO analysis of Department of Veterans Affairs (VA) data. | GAO-19-478.

Notes: Data reviewed included veterans who were authorized to use community care at least once in the fiscal year.

Figure 5. Number of Veterans Authorized to Use Community Care, Fiscal Years 2014 through 2018.

VA Updated Its Projection Model to Develop Most of Its Community Care Budget Estimate; Subsequent Changes Reflect More Current Information and Other Factors

VA first developed a separate budget estimate for community care to inform the President's fiscal year 2017 budget request. Beginning with the President's fiscal year 2018 budget request, VA updated its EHCPM to develop over 75 percent of its community care budget estimate and used other methods to develop the remainder. Subsequent changes were made to the community care budget estimates developed by the EHCPM for fiscal years 2018 and 2019 through successively higher levels of review in VA and OMB.

VA First Developed a Separate Budget Estimate for Community Care as Part of the President's Fiscal Year 2017 Budget Request for VA

VA first developed a separate budget estimate of the resources it would need for community care—as distinct from the care provided in VA medical facilities—in order to inform the President's fiscal year 2017 budget request for VA. Prior to this fiscal year 2017 budget request, VA developed a single budget estimate of the resources needed to provide all VA health care services, regardless of whether these services were purchased from community providers or delivered in VA medical facilities, because all these services were to be funded through the same appropriation account.[37] According to VA officials, at the time a separate community care appropriation account and budget estimate were unnecessary, because community care accounted for a relatively small portion of VA's overall health care budget. However, once the medical community care appropriation account was established in fiscal year 2017, VA began developing a separate budget estimate for community care, as required by law.[38]

To develop its first estimate of the resources needed for community care for fiscal year 2017, VA made adjustments to existing estimates for total demand for care—both in VA medical facilities and community care combined—developed by the EHCPM. At the time, VA used the EHCPM to estimate the resources needed to provide VA health care services to veterans, including inpatient, outpatient, and long-term care. However, the EHCPM did not make separate estimates for community care and care

[37] Community care services were funded, in part, through the Veterans Choice Fund during fiscal years 2015 and 2016. VA's health care budget estimates for those fiscal years did not include estimates for the Choice Program due to the timing of the implementation of the Choice Program in relation timing to the budget process.

[38] Pub. L. No. 114-41, § 4003, 129 Stat. 443, 462-463 (2015).

provided at VA facilities; according to VA officials, VA adjusted the EHCPM estimates by assuming that for each service, the share of total utilization and costs devoted to community care would be the same as they had been in the most recently completed fiscal year. In addition, after this adjustment, VA made additional changes to the community care budget estimate, which resulted in a net increase of $2.5 billion. Nearly all of this increase reflected an anticipated impact of the expanded access under the Choice Program, according to VA officials. Overall, this approach accounted for about 75 percent of the $12.3 billion community care budget estimate that informed the President's budget request for fiscal year 2017.

To develop the remaining portion of its community care budget estimate, VA used methods other than the EHCPM that, according to VA officials, were used historically to develop estimates of the resources needed for the state home per diem program and benefit programs. For example, VA develops budget estimates for certain services under the state home per diem program by creating projections of the amount of care to be provided using information about the size and demographic characteristics of the enrolled veteran population and projections of the unit cost of providing one day of care using recent cost experience.

According to VA officials, VA was able to continue using these other methods, because the services under these programs have been provided through community providers and not VA medical facilities. While methods for each program vary, in general, these methods are based on each program's historical utilization and costs. (See app. II for additional information on the methods VA uses to develop the budget estimates for each of these community care programs.)

Beginning with the President's Fiscal Year 2018 Budget Request, VA Updated Its Projection Model to Develop over 75 Percent of Its Community Care Budget Estimate

Beginning with the President's fiscal year 2018 budget request, VA updated its EHCPM directly to estimate most of the resources needed to purchase community care for veterans. Specifically, VA updated the EHCPM to estimate the amount of resources needed to purchase a set of more than 40 community care services that have accounted for over 75 percent of VA's total community care budget estimates of $12.6 billion for fiscal year 2018 and $12.4 billion for fiscal year 2019.[39]

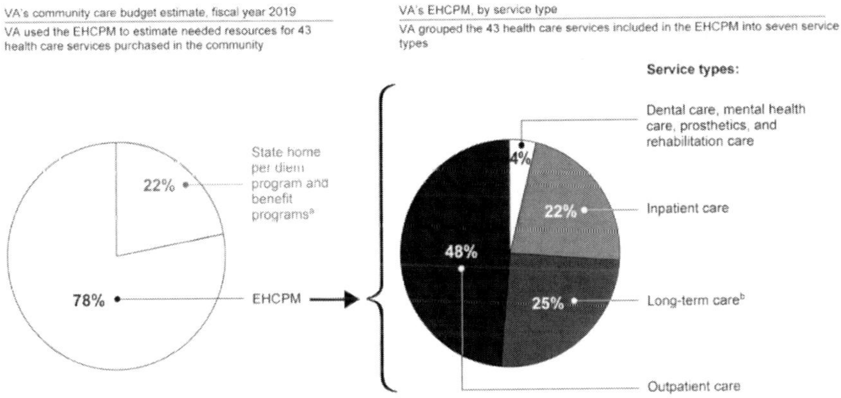

Source: GAO analysis of VA information. | GAO-19-478.

Note: Percentages may not sum to 100 due to rounding.

[a]State home per diem program includes adult day care, home domiciliary, and nursing care provided to veterans through state homes for eligible veterans. Benefit programs include the Civilian Health and Medical Program of the Department of Veterans Affairs, as well as other benefit programs that provide care for veterans and other eligible beneficiaries, such as spouses and dependent children, through community providers.

[b]Long-term care includes nursing home care in community nursing homes and home and community- based care, such as, community adult day care, homemaker/home health aide, home hospice and palliative care; purchased skilled home care and respite care.

Figure 6. Proportion of Department of Veterans Affairs (VA) Community Care Budget Estimate Developed Using VA's Enrollee Health Care Projection Model (EHCPM), by Service Type, Fiscal Year 2019.

---

[39] According to VA officials, these approximately 40 services were the health care services that were available to veterans in the community.

These health care services were grouped into seven service types and include outpatient care, inpatient care, and long-term care. (See app. III for a list of the health care services). Of these services, outpatient services typically accounted for the largest share of VA's community care budget estimate. For the remainder of community care services—including services provided under the state home per diem program and benefit programs— VA did not use the EHCPM and instead continued to use the other methods it has historically used to develop budget estimates for these services. (See Figure 6.)

VA made several changes to the EHCPM to develop most of its community care budget estimate. Historically, the EHCPM estimated resources needed to meet the total expected demand for VA health care—a combination of care provided in VA medical facilities and through community care programs. VA updated the EHCPM to determine the proportion of demand met by community care by projecting enrolled veterans' expected utilization of community care and the expected costs of purchasing these services.[40] In what follows, we describe five major changes made to the EHCPM allowing VA to estimate the budgetary resources needed for community care.

- Reliance on community care services. The EHCPM has historically accounted for the extent to which enrolled veterans would be projected to obtain health care services through the VA as opposed to other health care programs or insurers—referred to as reliance on VA health care.[41] VA updated the EHCPM so that it can further account for the extent to which enrolled veterans would be expected to use VA's community care programs as opposed to using care in VA's medical facilities. Each year, the EHCPM

[40] To estimate likely utilization and costs of community care, the EHCPM relies on several different data sources, including claims data from the Choice Program and other community care programs. (See app. IV, which describes the various data sources used.)

[41] VA estimates that at least 80 percent of veterans that have enrolled in VA health care have some type of public or private health care coverage other than VA. Many enrolled veterans use VA for some of their health care needs, but choose their other health care coverage for the rest. Because VA does not provide for 100 percent of the health care needs of enrolled veterans, this reduces the number of services required from VA.

determines reliance on VA community care based on a combination of historical experience—or the extent to which community care was used in prior fiscal years— and on the projected impact of new VA policies and operational guidance. For example, for the fiscal year 2019 budget estimates, the EHCPM projected reliance on VA care to be about 38 percent, of which 14 percent would be met through community care. Thus, the EHCPM projected reliance on VA's community care programs to be about 5.3 percent for all care enrolled veterans are projected to use in fiscal year 2019.[42]

- Accounting for difference in community providers' efficiency delivering inpatient services. VA also updated the EHCPM so that community care utilization projections account for the fact that veterans receiving inpatient care through community providers generally have relatively shorter lengths of inpatient stays compared with veterans receiving care at VA medical facilities.[43] According to officials from VA and its actuarial consultant, community providers on average have historically performed better than VA providers on national benchmarks measuring how well providers manage the length of inpatient stays, while not affecting quality of care. To account for this difference, VA uses an adjustment factor when projecting utilization of inpatient services based on potentially avoidable days of care for community providers.[44]
- Comparing projected utilization with actual utilization for community care services. VA developed an adjustment factor for the EHCPM's utilization estimates to account specifically for the

[42] To project fiscal year 2019 budget estimates, VA used fiscal year 2016 data to determine reliance on community care. VA's reliance on community care services may change once VA finalizes the new access standards under the VA MISSION Act, which bases eligibility on average drive times and wait times, among other factors.

[43] Historically, EHCPM utilization projections have reflected a combination of the length of inpatient stays for community providers and VA facilities, according to VA officials.

[44] For example, if the national benchmark length of stay is 5 days of care for an inpatient surgery and 30 percent of those 5 days are avoidable, the length of a "well managed" stay is 3.5 days. The adjustment factor reflects the historical level of performance for community providers relative to a well-managed stay.

differences between projected utilization and actual utilization of community care for the most recently completed fiscal year of data.[45] According to VA officials, the difference typically reflects utilization behavior among providers or patients that are difficult to estimate based solely on historical data—such as changes in local practice patterns (e.g., providers choosing to use magnetic resonance imaging versus x-rays).[46] To account for this behavior, VA compares projected and actual utilization and creates an "actual-to-expected" adjustment factor for each health care service to account for the difference.[47]

- Projecting unit costs for community care services. VA updated the EHCPM so that it could estimate what are known as the unit costs of purchasing community care services for veterans.[48] In general, the unit cost of a community care service comprises the payment made to the provider (known as direct patient costs), as well as the indirect costs associated with administration and overhead. Indirect costs include (1) the fees paid to the contractors for administrative responsibilities for the Choice Program, (2) VA billing and processing costs and care coordination costs associated community care programs, and (3) certain costs associated with the VA Central Office that support community care (e.g., the salaries for officials from the Office of Community Care and other VA Central Office officials).[49]

---

[45] Historically, VA has compared the EHCPM's projected utilization of all VA health care services—both delivered in VA facilities and community care—with actual utilization in the most recently completed fiscal year.

[46] This unexplained utilization is the net impact of a number of factors that often cannot be identified or quantified, including unique local practice patterns, evolving practice patterns or programs, coding issues, capacity constraints, and/or limitations in the data used to measure morbidity and reliance, or other model factors.

[47] For example, if the actual utilization for a service was determined to be 5 percent lower than the projected, the factor used for the actual-to-expected adjustment would be 0.95.

[48] Unit costs are costs to VA of purchasing a unit of service, such as an outpatient office visit or a day of care at an inpatient community facility.

[49] The Agency for Healthcare Research and Quality defines care coordination as the practice of organizing patient care activities and sharing information among all of the participants concerned with a patient's care to achieve safer, more effective care. Participants may share clinical data using manual methods such as faxing paper records, but these methods can be time-consuming and costly. Information technology has the potential to improve the

- Accounting for community care service complexity and inflation. VA made other changes to the EHCPM's unit cost projections for community care. For example, VA updated the EHCPM so that it accounts for costs associated with changes in the complexity—that is, the level of resources required to deliver—of health care services VA purchases from community providers. Officials from VA and its actuarial consultant noted that more complex services require relatively more resources to deliver, such as more expensive equipment (e.g., magnetic resonance imaging); more provider time; or higher-cost providers, such as surgeons. Officials anticipate that most services that VA purchases in the community will increase in complexity, leading to higher projected unit-costs for community care.[50] VA also updated the EHCPM so that its unit cost estimates for community care account for inflation in the cost of labor and equipment.

VA's Community Care Budget Estimates Projected by the Model for Fiscal Years 2018 and 2019 Were Subsequently Changed to Reflect More Current Information, among Other Factors

VA's community care budget estimates are reviewed at successively higher levels at VA and OMB to inform the President's budget request for VA.

---

efficiency of care coordination by allowing VA, the Choice Program third-party administrators, community providers, and veterans to electronically exchange information for care coordination purposes.

[50] According to officials from VA and its actuarial consultant, changes in the complexity of care can occur for a variety of reasons including the development of new drug therapies that replace less effective, less expensive therapies, such as the hepatitis C treatments that have become available in recent years; and changes in health care practices, such as greater use of magnetic resonance imaging to diagnose a condition.

VA identified several changes made during the review process to its estimates projected by the EHCPM for fiscal years 2018 and 2019; these changes were due to the availability of more current information related to utilization and costs, among other factors.

For fiscal year 2018, changes resulted in a budget request for VA community care in the President's budget request that was approximately $1 billion lower than VA's original EHCPM budget estimate of $10.7 billion.[51] These changes included the following:

- A $996 million decrease reflecting the availability of more current information showing that an anticipated increase in utilization due to the Choice Program was too high.[52]
- A $600 million decrease reflecting the availability of more current information showing that overhead costs initially allocated to community care in the data used in the EHCPM were too high.
- A $180 million decrease accounting for VA's implementation of a new law that reduces VHA's use of community care for examinations determining veterans' disability ratings.[53]
- A $500 million increase accounting for a court ruling that affected veteran eligibility for reimbursement of emergency community care, which was expected to increase utilization.[54]
- A $250 million increase reflecting the availability of more current information that indicated administrative costs for the Choice Program in the data used in the EHCPM were too low.

For fiscal year 2019, changes resulted in a budget request for VA community care in the President's budget request that was nearly $1 billion

---

[51] VA estimated $12.6 billion in total community care obligations for fiscal year 2018.
[52] According to VA officials, the anticipated increase in community care utilization was specifically related to veterans who were eligible for the Choice Program because the next available medical appointment with a VA provider was more than 30 days away.
[53] See 38 U.S.C. § 5101 note.
[54] Staab v. McDonald, 28 Vet. App. 50 (2016).

higher than VA's original EHCPM budget estimate of $8.6 billion.[55] These changes included the following:

- A $1.7 billion increase reflecting more current information indicating that community care administrative costs and the utilization levels in the data used in the EHCPM were too low.
- A $1 billion increase accounting for a delay in the timing of the implementation of community care network contracts. According to VA officials, this resulted in the continued use of reimbursement rates in community care that were higher than Medicare reimbursement rates.[56]
- A $1.8 billion decrease that reflected VA's implementation of a new policy that changed the timing of community care obligations from when a veteran is authorized to use community care to the when a claim for actual services is paid.

VA's Actual Obligations for Community Care in Fiscal Years 2017 and 2018 Were Higher than Estimated and Included Additional Funding Received for the Choice Program

VA's Actual Obligations for Community Care in Fiscal Years 2017 and 2018 Were $1.2 Billion and $2.2 Billion Higher than Estimated, Respectively

Our analysis of data included in VA's budget justifications shows that in fiscal years 2017 and 2018, VA obligated $1.2 billion and $2.2 billion

[55] VA estimated $12.4 billion in total community care obligations for fiscal year 2019.

[56] According to officials, VA included in the EHCPM anticipated savings from VA transitioning to Medicare reimbursement rates.

more for community care than originally estimated at the time of the President's budget requests for those years.[57] In both years, VA's actual obligations for both the Choice Program and other community care programs were higher than estimated (See Table 3).

Table 3. Department of Veterans Affairs' actual and estimated community care obligations, fiscal years 2017 and 2018

	Obligations (dollars in billions)					
Program	Fiscal year 2017			Fiscal year 2018		
	Actual	Estimated	Difference	Actual	Estimated	Difference
Veterans Choice Program	5.5	4.8	0.7	4.5	3.5	1
Other community care programs	8.1	7.5	0.6	10.3	9.1	1.2
Total community care	13.6	12.3	1.2	14.9	12.6	2.2

Source: GAO analysis of Department of Veterans Affairs (VA) budget justification and VA data. | GAO-19-478.

Notes: Numbers may not sum to totals or differences due to rounding. Estimated obligations are developed months prior to the start of a fiscal year. In addition to services for veterans, other community care programs include the community care services that VA purchases for other eligible beneficiaries, which may include a veteran's spouse or dependent child.

According to VA officials, the higher-than-estimated obligations for the Choice Program for fiscal year 2017 were driven, in part, due to changes in Choice Program policies and a large increase in the cost per authorization for care.[58]

---

[57] For fiscal years 2017 and 2018, we examined data for community care obligations for the Veterans Choice Fund and the Medical Community Care appropriation account. For comparison purposes, VA's budget justifications also show that in fiscal years 2017 and 2018, VA obligated $2.5 billion and $1.2 billion less for services provided in VA medical facilities than originally estimated at the time of the President's budget requests for those years. VA's actual obligations for these services totaled $59.4 and $62.9 billion for fiscal years 2017 and 2018, respectively.

[58] For example, VA made a policy change in June 2017, by issuing a policy memorandum that directed VA medical facilities to refer veterans to the Choice Program only if they met wait-time, distance, and geographic eligibility criteria, and to instead use other VA medical facilities, other facilities with which VA has sharing agreements, and other community care programs to deliver care to veterans when services were not available at a VA medical

Table 4. Comparison of Department of Veterans Affairs' actual and estimated obligations for selected community care service types, fiscal year 2017

	Obligations (dollars in millions). Fiscal year 2017		
Selected service type	Actual[a]	Estimated	Difference
Outpatient care	4,658	3,782	875
Inpatient care	3,016	2,656	360
CHAMPVA and other benefit programs' services[b]	1,290	1,697	(407)
Non-institutional care[c]	1,248	1,436	(188)
Community nursing home	870	1,012	(143)

Source: GAO analysis of Department of Veterans Affairs (VA) budget justification and VA data. | GAO-19-478.

Notes: This table includes service types that had a difference of $90 million or more between actual and estimated obligations. Differences reflect rounding. Estimated obligations are developed months prior to the start of a fiscal year. For fiscal year 2017, data reflect community care obligations for the Veterans Choice Fund and the Medical Community Care appropriation account.

[a]According to VA officials, the actual obligation amounts for certain service types for fiscal year 2017 were understated due to the way adjustments were accounted for in VA's financial management system. The adjustment was $700 million in fiscal year 2017.

[b]The Civilian Health and Medical Program of the Department of Veterans Affairs (CHAMPVA), as well as other benefit programs provide care for veterans and other eligible beneficiaries, such as spouses and dependent children, through community providers.

[c]Non-institutional care includes home and community-based long-term care programs, such as community adult day care, homemaker/home health aide programs, home hospice and palliative care, purchased skilled home care, and respite care.

In the case of other community care programs, VA officials told us that the higher-than-estimated obligations for both fiscal years 2017 and 2018 were driven, in part, by local practice patterns (e.g., providers choosing to use magnetic resonance imaging versus x-rays) and the capacity of VA medical facilities to provide services. As discussed later in this chapter, VA also received and reallocated additional funding to purchase

facility and veterans did not qualify under the Veterans Access, Choice, and Accountability Act's eligibility criteria. In August 2017, VA changed its guidance and issued a fact sheet directing VA medical facilities to refer veterans to the Choice Program to the maximum extent possible. See Department of Veterans Affairs, *Extension of Veterans Choice Program Funding,* VA Fact Sheet (Washington, D.C.: August 2017).

community care in fiscal years 2017 and 2018, which contributed to actual obligations being higher-than-estimated obligations.[59]

Table 5. Comparison of Department of Veterans Affairs' actual and estimated obligations for selected community care service types, fiscal year 2018

	Obligations (dollars in millions). Fiscal year 2018		
Selected service type	Actual[a]	Estimated	Difference
Outpatient care	4,287	3,545	742
Dental care	238	146	91
Inpatient care	2,649	3,104	(455)
CHAMPVA and other benefit programs' services[b]	1,345	1,649	(305)
Community nursing home	937	1,032	(96)

Source: GAO analysis of Department of Veterans Affairs (VA) budget justification and VA data. | GAO-19-478.

Notes: This table includes service types that had a difference of $90 million or more between actual and estimated obligations. Differences reflect rounding. Estimated obligations are developed months prior to the start of a fiscal year. For fiscal year 2018, data reflect community care obligations for the Veterans Choice Fund and the Medical Community Care appropriation account.

[a]According to VA officials, the actual obligation amounts for certain service types for fiscal year 2018 were understated due to the way adjustments were accounted for in VA's financial management system. These adjustments were $2.2 billion for fiscal year 2018.

[b]The Civilian Health and Medical Program of the Department of Veterans Affairs (CHAMPVA) as well as other benefit programs provide care for veterans and other eligible beneficiaries, such as spouses and dependent children, through community providers.

Our analysis of VA's obligations by service type shows that in fiscal year 2017, VA's higher-than-estimated obligations for community care were primarily for outpatient and inpatient services, as shown in table 4.[60] In fiscal year 2018, the higher-than-estimated obligations for community

[59] In future work, we plan to review VA's development of its community care budget estimate, including how the department is incorporating lessons learned from its 2017 and 2018 estimates as it continues using the EHCPM for that purpose.

[60] According to VA officials, the actual obligation amounts for certain service types for fiscal years 2017 and 2018 were understated due to the way adjustments were accounted for in VA's financial management system. These adjustments were $700 million for fiscal year 2017 and $2.2 billion for fiscal year 2018. VA stated that they anticipate these adjustments to decrease starting in fiscal year 2019 as a result of a VA policy change regarding the timing of certain community care obligations.

care were primarily for outpatient services, while there was an overall decrease in obligations for inpatient services. (See table 5.) Additionally, for some service types, VA's actual obligations were lower than estimated in fiscal years 2017 and 2018.[61]

VA's Higher-Than-Estimated Obligations for Community Care Included Additional Funding VA Received for the Choice Program Outside of the Annual Appropriations Process

To obligate $13.6 billion for community care in fiscal year 2017 and $14.9 billion in fiscal year 2018—amounts that were $1.2 billion and $2.2 billion higher, respectively, than what VA originally estimated for its budget request, and what VA received in its annual appropriation—VA requested and received additional Choice Program funding outside of the annual appropriations process. VA also reallocated funding from other sources, including unobligated funding from a prior fiscal year and collections, to pay for the other community care programs.[62]

Specifically, the $13.6 billion and $14.9 billion VA obligated for community care in fiscal years 2017 and 2018, respectively, came from the following sources:

- Choice Program. For both fiscal years, VA obligated from its remaining funding and prior-year recoveries from the previous fiscal years, and requested and received additional funding three times outside of the annual appropriations process.[63] (Table 6

[61] For fiscal years 2017 and 2018, we examined data for community care obligations for the Veterans Choice Fund and the Medical Community Care appropriation account.

[62] Due to the nature of VA's multi-year authority in some of its appropriations, budget authority may be available from unobligated balances, which remain available for a fixed period of time in excess of one fiscal year. Collections refers to the resources VA expects to collect from health insurers of veterans who receive VA care for nonservice-connected conditions and other sources, such as veterans' copayments.

[63] Prior-year recoveries refers to obligations that were estimated for authorizations for the previous fiscal year, but were never liquidated. For fiscal year 2017, VA de-obligated around $700 million in Choice Program funds from fiscal year 2017 authorizations for use in 2018. For fiscal year 2018, this amount was around $295 million.

below summarizes the time frames during which VA requested and received additional appropriations for the Choice Program outside of the annual appropriations process for fiscal years 2017 and 2018.)

- Other community care programs. For both fiscal years, VA obligated from its annual appropriation and transferred a portion of its overall collections from its Medical Care Collections Fund to the medical community care account.[64] In addition, for fiscal year 2018, VA used unobligated funding and prior-year recoveries from fiscal year 2017.[65]

Table 6. Department of Veterans Affairs' Veterans Choice Program budget timeline, fiscal years 2017 and 2018

Date	Budget event
2016:	
February	The President submitted the fiscal year 2017 budget request to Congress, which included requested resources for VA health care. As the Veterans Choice Program (Choice Program) was expected to end in August 2017, VA estimated it would use its remaining $4.8 billion in Choice Program funding from fiscal year 2016. The Choice Program originally began with $10 billion in funding.[a]
September	Fiscal year 2017 appropriations for VA enacted.[b]
2017:	
April	Legislation enacted allowing the Choice Program to continue until funding for the program is exhausted regardless of time.[c]
May	The President submitted the fiscal year 2018 budget request to Congress. VA estimated it would use its remaining $626 million in available Choice Program funding from fiscal year 2017, and requested $2.9 billion in new Choice Program appropriations for fiscal year 2018.

[64] For fiscal years 2017 and 2018, VA was appropriated $7.2 billion and $419 million (in addition to advance appropriations of $9.4 billion), respectively, for its medical community care account. For fiscal year 2017, VA transferred $1.25 billion in collections from its Medical Care Collections Fund to its medical community care account, which was $1 billion higher than what VA initially estimated it would transfer at the time of the President's budget request. For fiscal year 2018, VA transferred about $272 million in collections.

[65] For fiscal year 2018, VA had $470 million in unobligated funding for its medical community care account from fiscal year 2017, and $256 million in prior year recoveries from fiscal year 2017.

Date	Budget event
June	The Secretary of Veterans Affairs testified at a congressional subcommittee hearing regarding VA's fiscal year 2018 budget request. During the testimony, the Secretary informed Congress that due to an increase in utilization, Choice Program funding would run out prior to September, the end of fiscal year 2017.
August	Legislation enacted that provided $2.1 billion in funding for the Choice Program.[d] According to VA, this amount was needed to maintain the program while the department worked to secure funding for the remainder of fiscal year 2018.
December	The Secretary informed Congress on December 12 that Choice Program funding would be exhausted in 3-to-5 weeks.
	Legislation enacted on December 22 provided $2.1 billion in funding for the Choice Program.[e]
2018:	
March	The Secretary testified at a congressional subcommittee hearing regarding VA's fiscal year 2019 budget request. During the testimony, the Secretary informed Congress that as of March 16, about $1.1 billion remained of the $2.1 billion in funds appropriated in December 2017, and that funding would be exhausted before the end of fiscal year 2018.
	Fiscal year 2018 appropriations for VA enacted.[f] It did not include any additional appropriations for the Choice Program.
May	The Acting Secretary of Veterans Affairs sent a letter to Congress stating that the Choice Program would run out of funding by the end of the month.
June	Legislation enacted that provided $5.2 billion in funding for the Choice Program.[g] This funding was expected to keep the Choice Program operating until VA's new community care program goes into effect, which was expected to be by June 2019.
October	Start of fiscal year 2019.

Source: GAO analysis. | GAO-19-478.

[a]At the time of the Department of Veterans Affairs' (VA) fiscal year 2017 budget justification, VA estimated there was $4.8 billion in funding for the Choice Program. However, VA's fiscal year 2019 budget justification shows only $4.4 billion in Choice Program funding for fiscal year 2017. The Veterans Access, Choice, and Accountability Act of 2014 provided $10 billion in funding for the Choice Program, which was implemented in early fiscal year 2015 and authorized until funds were exhausted or through August 7, 2017, whichever occurred first. Pub. L. No. 113-146, §§ 101(p), 802, 128 Stat. 1754, 1763, 1802-1803 (2014).

[b]Pub.L. No. 114-223, tit. II, 130 Stat. 857, 867 (2016).

[c]Pub.L. No. 115-26, § 1, 131 Stat. 129 (2017).

[d]See VA Choice and Quality Employment Act of 2017, Pub. L. No. 115-46, § 101, 131 Stat. 958, 959 (2017).

[e]An act to amend the Homeland Security Act of 2002 to require the Secretary of Homeland Security to issue Department of Homeland Security-wide guidance and develop training programs as part of the Department of Homeland Security Blue Campaign, and for other purposes, Pub. L. No. 115-96. Div. D, § 4001, 131 Stat. 2044, 2052-53 (2017).

[f]Pub. L. No. 115-141, 132 Stat. 348 (2018).

[g]VA MISSION Act of 2018. Pub. L.No. 115-182, tit. I, 132 Stat. 1393 (2018).

Agency Comments

We provided a draft of this product to VA and OMB for comment. VA provided technical comments, which we incorporated as appropriate. OMB had no comments.

We are sending copies of this chapter to the Secretary of Veterans Affairs, the Director of the Office of Management and Budget, appropriate congressional committees, and other interested parties.

Sincerely yours,

Sharon M. Silas
Acting Director, Health Care

Appendix I: The Department of Veterans Affairs' Community Care Programs for Veterans and Other Eligible Beneficiaries

While the majority of veterans utilizing Department of Veterans Affairs' (VA) health care services receive care in VA-operated medical facilities, veterans may also obtain services from non-VA providers in the community—known as community care—through one of several community care programs aimed at helping to ensure that veterans receive timely and accessible care.[66] In implementing the VA MISSION Act, VA plans to consolidate four of its community care programs for veterans—dialysis contracts, individually authorized care, the Patient- Centered Community Care Program, and the Veterans Choice Program— under the Veterans Community Care Program, which is expected to go into effect by

[66] Unless otherwise indicated, the terms "community care" and "community providers" refer, respectively, to the services the department purchases outside VA medical facilities. Additionally, "community care programs" includes programs and activities that provide community care whether under statutory or contractual authority.

June 2019.[67] In addition, VA has several other community care programs that serve veterans and programs that provide health care services to other eligible beneficiaries, including a veteran's spouse or dependent child.

Community Care Programs for Veterans that VA Plans to Consolidate

Dialysis Contracts

When dialysis services—a life-saving medical procedure for patients with permanent kidney failure—are not feasibly available at VA medical facilities, veterans may be referred to one of VA's contracted dialysis providers, and veterans may receive dialysis at local clinics on an outpatient basis, or at home (if the contractors offer home- based dialysis services).

Individually Authorized Care

When a veteran cannot access a particular specialty care service from a VA medical facility—either because the service is not offered, the veteran would have to wait too long for an appointment, or the veteran would have to travel a long distance to a VA medical facility—VA medical facility staff may request an individual authorization for the veteran to obtain the service from a community provider who is willing to accept VA payment.

Patient-Centered Community Care

VA contracted with two third-party administrators to develop regional networks of community providers of specialty care, mental health care, limited emergency care, and maternity and limited newborn care when such care is not feasibly available from a VA medical facility. To be eligible to obtain care from Patient-Centered Community Care providers,

---

[67] John S. McCain III, Daniel K. Akaka, and Samuel R. Johnson VA Maintaining Internal Systems and Strengthening Integrated Outside Networks Act of 2018. Pub. L.No. 115- 182, tit. I, 132 Stat. 1392 (2018) (VA MISSION Act).

veterans must meet the same criteria that are required for individually authorized care.

Veterans Choice Program

VA modified its Patient-Centered Community Care contracts with the two third-party administrators to implement the Veterans Choice Program. This program allows eligible veterans to obtain health care services from community providers if the veteran meets certain criteria, including when a veteran cannot receive care within 30 days from the veteran's or physician's preferred date, or face an unusual or excessive burden in traveling to a VA medical center.[68]

Other Community Care Programs for Veterans

Agreements with Federal Partners and Academic Affiliates

When services are not available at VA medical facilities, VA may obtain specialty, inpatient, and outpatient health care services for veterans through different types of sharing agreements—those with other federal facilities (such as those operated by the Department of Defense and the Indian Health Service), those with Tribal Health Programs, and those with university-affiliated hospitals, medical schools, and practice groups (known as academic affiliates).

Emergency Care

When emergency community care is not preauthorized, VA may reimburse community providers for emergency care for eligible veterans

[68] Other criteria for the Veterans Choice Program include if the veteran lives more than 40 miles driving distance from the nearest VA medical center with a full-time primary care physician; or would have to travel by air, boat, or ferry to the VA medical center closest to their home; or have specific health care needs that warrant participation (including the nature and frequency of care); or live in a state or territory without a full-service VA medical center.

for a condition related to a service-connected disability, and for eligible veterans for a condition not related to a service- connected disability.[69]

Foreign Medical Program

The Foreign Medical Program is VA's health care benefits program for eligible veterans who are residing or traveling abroad and have a service-connected disability.

State Home Per Diem Program

Under the State Home Per Diem Program, states provide care for eligible veterans in three different types of programs: nursing home, domiciliary, and adult day health care.

Community Care Programs for Other Beneficiaries

Camp Lejeune Family Member Program

The Camp Lejeune Family Member Program is for family members of veterans that lived or served at U.S. Marine Corps Base Camp Lejeune, North Carolina, for no fewer than 30 days between January 1, 1957, and December 31, 1987, and were potentially exposed to drinking water contaminated with industrial solvents, benzene, and other chemicals. The program provides health care to veterans who served on active duty at Camp Lejeune and to reimburse eligible Camp Lejeune family members

[69] A veteran may access emergency care for a condition related to a service-connected disability when a prudent layperson (1) would classify the condition as an emergency, and (2) would have deemed it unreasonable for the veteran to access the care at a VA or other federal facility. In addition to meeting the previously stated criteria, a veteran may access emergency care for a condition not related to a service-connected disability if services were rendered before they were stable for transfer to a VA or other federal facility; if the veteran was enrolled in and accessed care from a VA clinician in the 24 months preceding the emergency care; if the veteran is financially liable to the community provider; if the veteran has no entitlement under another health plan contract (such as Medicare); and if the veteran has no recourse against a third party that would wholly extinguish liability to the community provider.

for health care costs related to one or more of 15 specified illnesses or medical conditions specified in law.[70]

Children of Women Vietnam Veterans Health Care Benefits Program

This program provides health care benefits to female Vietnam veterans' birth children who the Veterans Benefits Administration has determined to have a covered birth defect. This program is not a comprehensive health care plan and only covers those services necessary for the treatment of a covered birth defect and associated medical conditions.

Civilian Health and Medical Program of the Department of Veterans Affairs (CHAMPVA)

CHAMPVA is a comprehensive health care program that provides health care coverage for spouses, children and primary caregivers of veterans who are permanently and totally disabled from a service-connected disability.[71] CHAMPVA functions similarly to traditional health insurance, with most care in the program delivered using non-VA community providers.

Spina Bifida Health Care Benefits Program

This program provides health care benefits to certain Korea and Vietnam veterans' birth children who have been diagnosed with spina bifida.[72]

---

[70] Examples of conditions listed in the law include bladder cancer, breast cancer, leukemia, and lung cancer. See Pub. L. No. 112-154, § 102, 126 Stat. 1165 (2012).

[71] CHAMPVA also provides coverage for spouses and children of those who died in the line of duty or from a service-connected disability. Eligibility for spouses also includes widowed spouses. See 38 U.S.C. § 1781.

[72] Spina bifida is a type of birth defect that results from the neural tube (the embryonic structure that eventually develops into the brain and spinal cord) failing to develop or close properly in utero, which can cause a range of physical and neurological defects.

Appendix II: Budget Formulation Process for the State Home Per Diem Program and Non-Veteran Community Care Programs

The Department of Veterans Affairs (VA) and its actuarial consultant use the Enrollee Health Care Projection Model to develop most of the department's estimate of the resources needed to meet the expected demand for VA's health care services. VA uses other methods to estimate the remaining resources needed. This remaining portion includes community care programs for veterans and other eligible beneficiaries, including the State Home Per Diem Program and the Civilian Health and Medical Program of the Department of Veterans Affairs (CHAMPVA).[73]

State Home Per Diem Program

This program pays per diem for state- provided care for eligible veterans in three different types of programs: domiciliary, nursing home, and adult day health care. For state home domiciliary and nursing care, categorized as institutional care, VA creates budget projections based on historical funding data. For state home adult day health care, categorized as non-institutional care, VA's budget estimates are based on projections of the amount of care provided— which is known as workload—and the unit cost of providing a day of this care.[74] VA projects the demand for non-institutional care services using information about the size and demographic characteristics of the enrolled veteran population. VA projects unit cost for non-institutional care services by calculating unit-cost increases observed from recent experience and then using this information to project future unit costs. VA multiplies the workload estimates, unit-cost estimates, and the number of days in the fiscal year to develop an estimate of the amount of resources needed for non-institutional care.

---

[73] Other eligible beneficiaries may include a veteran's spouse or dependent child.

[74] Workload for most non-institutional services is measured as the average number of people enrolled per day for the number of days in the fiscal year that the service is available.

CHAMPVA

CHAMPVA provides health care coverage for spouses and children of veterans who are permanently and totally disabled from a service-connected disability.[75] CHAMPVA functions similarly to traditional health insurance—most care within CHAMPVA is delivered using non-VA community providers. Therefore, developing estimates of the resources needed for CHAMPVA requires factoring in utilization patterns and cost inflation that are generally outside of VA's control. Budget estimates for CHAMPVA are developed using a formula that computes the predicted number of users and costs per-member per-year.[76] VA works with its actuarial consultant to generate projections of CHAMPVA users that incorporate changes related to the population of disabled veterans and projections of expected increases and decreases in the CHAMPVA-eligible population. In addition, the actuarial consultant projects the costs per-member per-year, which is calculated by dividing the most current fiscal year data on total CHAMPVA expenditures by the number of actual users. Trends are then incorporated to predict the future costs per- member per-year, which is multiplied by projections of the number of CHAMPVA users to develop CHAMPVA budget estimates.

APPENDIX III: HEALTH CARE SERVICES INCLUDED IN THE ENROLLEE HEALTH CARE PROJECTION MODEL FOR FISCAL YEAR 2019

Using its Enrollee Health Care Projection Model (EHCPM), the Department of Veterans Affairs (VA) developed estimates for 79 health care services—available in VA medical facilities or through community care—for the fiscal year 2019 President's budget request. As shown in

---

[75] CHAMPVA also provides coverage for spouses and children of those who died in the line of duty or from a service-connected disability. Eligibility for spouses also includes widowed spouses. See 38 U.S.C. § 1781.

[76] VA considers members to be those who access CHAMPVA services.

Table 7, VA developed separate estimates for the 43 services that were available through community care. Some of these 43 services were only available through community care. These services were primarily long-term care, including nursing home care provided at community nursing homes, home hospice care, home respite care, homemaker or home health aid programs, and purchased skilled nursing care.

Table 7. Health care services included in the Department of Veterans Affairs' enrollee Health Care Projection Model, fiscal year 2019

Service type	Health care service	Estimates developed for VA facility care	Estimates developed for community care
Dental care			
	Major restorative dental services	checked	checked
	Minor restorative dental services	checked	checked
	Preventative and basic dental services	checked	checked
Inpatient care			
	Maternity deliveries	checked	checked
	Maternity non-deliveries	checked	checked
	Medical	checked	checked
	Surgical	checked	checked
Long-term care			
	Community adult day health care	N/A	checked
	Community nursing home (long stay)	N/A	checked
	Community nursing home (short stay)	N/A	checked
	Community residential care	checked	N/A
	Home-based primary care	checked	N/A
	Home hospice care	N/A	checked
	Home respite care	N/A	checked
	Homemaker/home health aide programs	N/A	checked
	Home telehealth	checked	N/A
	Purchased skilled home care	N/A	checked
	Spinal cord injury and disorders home care	checked	N/A

Table 7. (Continued)

Service type	Health care service	Estimates developed for VA facility care	Estimates developed for community care
	VA adult day health care	checked	N/A
	VA community living center (long stay)	checked	N/A
	VA community living center (short stay)	checked	N/A
Mental health care			
	Acute substance abuse	checked	checked
	Compensated work therapy/transitional residence	checked	N/A
	Homeless	checked	N/A
	Inpatient mental health	checked	checked
	Intensive community mental health recovery services	checked	N/A
	Mental health residential rehabilitation	checked	N/A
	Mental health office visits	checked	N/A
	Mental health residential rehabilitation treatment program outpatient encounters	checked	N/A
	Mental health residential rehabilitation treatment program residential encounters	checked	N/A
	Outpatient mental health	checked	checked
	Outpatient substance abuse	checked	checked
	Psychosocial rehabilitation and recovery centers	checked	N/A
	Psychotherapy (individual or group)	checked	checked
	Sustained treatment and rehabilitation	checked	checked
	Work therapy	checked	N/A
Outpatient care			
	Allergy immunotherapy	checked	checked
	Allergy testing	checked	checked
	Ambulance	N/A	checked
	Cardiovascular	checked	checked
	Chiropractic	checked	checked
	Compensation and pension exams	checked	N/A
	Dialysis and related services	checked	checked

Service type	Health care service	Estimates developed for VA facility care	Estimates developed for community care
Outpatient care			
	Emergency room visits	checked	checked
	Hearing aid services	checked	checked
	Hearing and speech exams	checked	checked
	Immunizations	checked	checked
	Maternity	checked	checked
	Miscellaneous medical	checked	checked
	Nutritional counseling	checked	checked
	Office administered drugs	checked	checked
	Office visits, urgent care, physical exams–non- mental health	checked	checked
	Outpatient medication therapy management	checked	checked
	Over-the-counter medication	checked	N/A
	Pathology	checked	checked
	Physical medicine	checked	checked
	Prescription drugs (brand and generic)	checked	N/A
	Prescription related supplies	checked	N/A
	Prosthetic and orthotic services	checked	checked
	Radiology—computerized tomography, magnetic resonance imaging, and positron emission tomography	checked	checked
	Radiology—general	checked	checked
	Recreational therapy	checked	N/A
	Surgery	checked	checked
	Vision exams	checked	checked
Prosthetics			
	Blind aids	checked	N/A
	Cardiothoracic surgical implants	checked	N/A
	Glasses/contacts	checked	N/A
	Hearing aids	checked	N/A
	Home telehealth devices	checked	N/A
	Medical equipment and supplies	checked	N/A
	Orthotics	checked	N/A
	Oxygen	checked	N/A
	Prosthetics-artificial limbs	checked	N/A

Table 7. (Continued)

Service type	Health care service	Estimates developed for VA facility care	Estimates developed for community care
	Respiratory equipment	checked	N/A
	Surgical implants	checked	N/A
	VA specialized products and services	checked	N/A
	Wheeled mobility devices	checked	N/A
Rehabilitation care			
	Blind rehabilitation	checked	N/A
	Spinal cord injury and disorders	checked	N/A

Source: GAO analysis of Department of Veterans Affairs (VA) data and documentation of the Enrollee Health Care Projection Model. | GAO-19-478.

Appendix IV: Community Care Data Sources in the Department of Veterans Affairs' Enrollee Health Care Projection Model

The Department of Veterans Affairs (VA) and its actuarial consultant use the Enrollee Health Care Projection Model (EHCPM) to develop most of the department's budget estimate to meet the expected demand for VA's health care services.[77] This estimate includes the services that VA purchases from non-VA community providers through its various community care programs, including the Veterans Choice Program (Choice Program).

[77] The EHCPM was developed in 1998 by VA and its actuarial consultant. VA uses other methods to estimate the remaining resources needed.

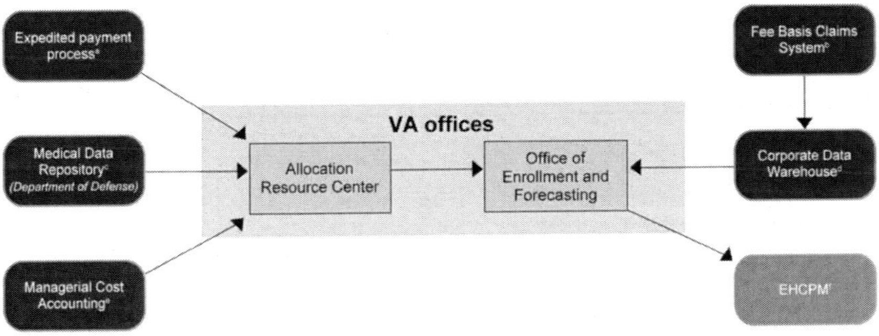

Source: GAO analysis of interviews with VA officials. | GAO-19-478.

[a]When the Veterans Choice Program was implemented in November 2014, all Veterans Choice Program claims were initially processed through the Fee Basis Claims System. In fiscal year 2016, due to Veterans Choice Program claim processing backlogs, some Veterans Choice Program claims were processed in an expedited manner outside of the Fee Basis Claims System from March 2016 through July 2016. These claims were aggregated and processed in bulk

[b]The Fee Basis Claims System processes claims for the Department of Veterans Affairs' (VA) community care programs nationwide at individual VA medical facilities and consolidated payment processing centers.

[c]The Allocation Resource Center pulled data from the Medical Data Repository on dual eligible veterans, or those veterans that are also eligible for medical benefits from the Department of Defense.

[d]VA's Corporate Data Warehouse is a national repository comprising data from several VA clinical and administrative systems.

[e]The Allocation Resource Center pulled indirect costs from VA's Managerial Cost Accounting system. Indirect costs include those costs associated with care coordination or claims processing.

[f]VA's Enrollee Health Care Projection Model (EHCPM) is operated by VA's actuarial consultant.

Figure 7. Data Sources for the Department of Veterans Affairs' 2017 Enrollee Health Care Projection Model.

Based on our interviews with various VA officials, VA's Office of Enrollment and Forecasting provided utilization and cost data from fiscal year 2016 community care claims from four different sources for use in the 2017 EHCPM, which was used to project the fiscal year 2019 budget estimate.[78] (See Figure 7). Specifically, the Office of Enrollment and Forecasting—which is responsible for compiling the claims data used in the EHCPM—obtained community care claims data, including Choice Program claims, from VA's Fee Basis Claims System. In addition, the Office of Enrollment and Forecasting worked with VA's Allocation Resource Center to gather additional utilization and cost data from Choice Program claims processed outside the Fee Basis Claims System, and other data needed for the 2017 EHCPM.[79] Specifically, the Allocation Resource Center compiled claims data for those Choice Program claims paid through expedited payments.[80] The Allocation Resource Center also pulled data on

---

[78] According to VA officials, they conduct risk assessments and review security controls of their financial management systems, including a recent review of the Fee Basis Claims System, to support the Secretary for Veterans Affairs' annual attestation of the effectiveness of internal control over those systems. In particular, the Secretary is responsible for establishing and maintaining effective internal controls and financial management systems that meet the objectives of 31 U.S.C. § 3512(c), (d), commonly known as the Federal Managers' Financial Integrity Act of 1982 and the Office of Management and Budget (OMB) Circular No. A 123, *Management's Responsibility for Enterprise Risk Management and Internal Control.* These objectives are to ensure (1) effective and efficient operations, (2) compliance with applicable laws and regulations, and (3) reliable financial reporting. The Federal Managers' Financial Integrity Act of 1982 and OMB Circular No. A-123 require an annual statement of assurance to Congress attesting to the effectiveness of internal controls and identifying material weaknesses. This statement is included as part of the VA's Agency Financial Report, which is published annually by November 15.

[79] According to VA officials, prior to the implementation of the Choice Program in November 2014, staff from the Office of Enrollment and Forecasting were responsible for pulling all relevant claims data needed by its actuarial consultant for the EHCPM. Because of the introduction of the Choice Program, and the changing ways through which Choice Program claims were processed, VA officials stated that the Office of Enrollment and Forecasting asked for assistance from the Allocation Resource Center to identify and gather Choice Program claims data. VA officials anticipate that once the Choice Program ends, staff from the Office of Enrollment and Forecasting will be responsible again for pulling the relevant claims data needed by its actuarial consultant for the EHCPM.

[80] Since implementation of the Choice Program in November 2014, VA has modified the way it has processed and paid Choice Program claims. All Choice Program claims were initially processed through the Fee Basis Claims System. Due to Choice Program claim processing backlogs, some Choice Program claims were processed in an expedited manner outside of the Fee Basis Claims System from March 2016 through July 2016. These claims were aggregated and processed in bulk. Since April 2017, VA has been processing Choice Program claims through a different claims processing system, Plexis Claims Manager. However, according to VA officials, a small number of Choice Program claims continue to be paid through an expedited payment process based on the date of service of the claim. For more information on changes to how Choice Program claims have been processed and paid, see Department of Veterans Affairs, Office of Inspector General, *Veterans Health Administration: Audit of the Timeliness and Accuracy of Choice Payments Processed Through the Fee Basis Claims System,* Report No. 15-03036-47 (Washington, D.C.: Dec.

dual eligible veterans, from the Department of Defense's Medical Data Repository, and indirect costs associated community care claims (for example, costs associated with care coordination or claims processing) from VA's Managerial Cost Accounting system.[81]

12, 2017), and Department of Veterans Affairs, Office of Inspector General, *Veterans Health Administration: Bulk Payments Made under Patient- Centered Community Care/Veterans Choice Program Contracts,* Report No. 17-02713- 231 (Washington, D.C.: Sept. 6, 2018).

[81] Dual eligible veterans are those veterans that are also eligible for medical benefits from the Department of Defense.

In: Key Government Reports. Volume 26 ISBN: 978-1-53616-568-5
Editor: Ernest Clark

Chapter 4

VETERANS HEALTH ADMINISTRATION: REGIONAL NETWORKS NEED IMPROVED OVERSIGHT AND CLEARLY DEFINED ROLES AND RESPONSIBILITIES*

United States Government Accountability Office

ABBREVIATIONS

FTE	full-time equivalent
SAIL	Strategic Analytics for Improvement and Learning
VA	Department of Veterans Affairs
VHA	Veterans Health Administration
VISN	Veterans Integrated Service Network

* This is an edited, reformatted and augmented accessible version of the United States Government Accountability Office Report to Congressional Requesters, Publication No. GAO-19-462, dated June 2019.

Why GAO Did This Study

VHA operates one of the nation's largest health care systems with 18 regional networks—VISNs—that manage and oversee 172 medical centers within defined geographic areas. VHA expects to provide care to more than 7 million veterans in fiscal year 2019, and demand for its services is expected to grow over time.

GAO was asked to conduct a review of VISNs, including VHA's oversight of VISNs. This chapter examines (1) the extent to which VHA oversees VISNs' management and oversight of medical centers and (2) how VHA oversees VISN staffing.

GAO reviewed VHA policies, guidance, and staffing data regarding VISNs. GAO also interviewed officials from VHA, all 18 VISNs, and four medical centers selected for variation in geography, urban or rural location, and complexity.

What GAO Recommends

GAO recommends that VHA (1) develop a process to assess the overall performance of VISNs in managing and overseeing medical centers, (2) establish a comprehensive policy that clearly defines VISN roles and responsibilities for managing and overseeing medical centers and (3) establish a process to routinely oversee VISN staffing. VHA concurred with the first and third recommendations, and concurred in principle with the second.

What GAO Found

The Veterans Health Administration's (VHA) oversight of its regional health care networks is limited. Within VHA, these networks—known as Veterans Integrated Service Networks (VISN)—manage the day-to-day functions of medical centers and also provide administrative and clinical oversight of medical centers. VHA's approach for overseeing VISNs does not include an assessment of each VISN as a whole. Instead, to assess VISN operations, VHA primarily relies on performance assessments of individual VISN directors, which are based in part on medical center performance data. VHA officials acknowledged that a VISN director's individual performance is not always indicative of the VISN's performance as a whole. VHA supplements these assessments with periodic meetings with VISN leadership, including quarterly reviews on specific topics, such as patient quality assurance metrics and best practices. However, GAO found that these quarterly reviews do not typically include discussion of VISN level performance measures, or how VISNs manage and oversee medical centers. By establishing a process for assessing the overall performance of VISNs in managing and overseeing medical centers, VHA would be better able to determine if a VISN's performance is positive, if it is functioning poorly, or if it requires remediation.

VHA also lacks a comprehensive policy to define VISN roles and responsibilities. VHA and VISN officials told GAO they have several documents they believe help VISNs understand these roles and responsibilities. However, these documents either focus on specific policies and programs, or are tied to individuals. The lack of clearly defined roles and responsibilities at the VISN level makes it difficult for VHA to develop an effective oversight process that ensures adequate monitoring of VISN activities.

VHA primarily oversees VISN staffing by using standardized staffing levels and positions, but does not ensure VISNs adhere to them. VHA has a standardized VISN organizational chart, which includes recommended staffing levels for each of the 18 VISNs—63 to 66 full-time-equivalent staff—and 28 key positions, including a chief medical officer and mental health lead, to be in place at each VISN. VHA officials told GAO they expect VISNs to adhere to the standardized chart, and that they conducted a one-time review that included checking that VISNs' total full-time equivalents were within the allotted allowance.

However, VHA's review did not ensure that VISN organizational charts always included the 28 key positions on the standardized chart. GAO found one to five key positions were not listed on the organizational charts of more than a third of VISNs, among those with organizational charts that VHA had reviewed and approved. For example, one VISN was missing the primary care and geriatrics and extended care positions on its organizational chart. VISN officials provided various reasons for the positions not being listed on the organizational charts, including that these responsibilities were being performed as a collateral duty for VISN or medical center staff. Without effective oversight, VHA leadership cannot provide reasonable assurance that VISNs are appropriately staffed, which may hinder.

RECOMMENDATIONS FOR EXECUTIVE ACTION

We are making the following three recommendations to the Department of Veterans Affairs:

- The Under Secretary for Health should develop a process to assess the overall performance of VISNs in managing and overseeing medical centers. (Recommendation 1)
- The Under Secretary for Health should establish a comprehensive policy that clearly defines VISN roles and responsibilities for managing and overseeing medical centers. (Recommendation 2)
- The Under Secretary for Health should establish a process to routinely oversee VISN staffing, to include ensuring VISNs are consistent with VHA's standardized VISN staffing levels and positions, and documenting the rationale for approving staffing that does not adhere to VHA's standardized approach. (Recommendation 3)

INTRODUCTION

June 19, 2019

The Veterans Health Administration (VHA), within the Department of Veterans Affairs (VA), operates one of the nation's largest health care systems, with 18 Veterans Integrated Service Networks (VISN) that manage and oversee 172 medical centers and other medical facilities. VHA anticipates that it will provide care to more than 7 million veterans in fiscal year 2019 and that demand for its services will grow in the coming years.

We and others have identified challenges VHA faces in managing and overseeing its health care system, including VHA's ability to ensure that its medical centers provide timely access to quality health care for veterans. These challenges contributed to VA health care's addition to GAO's High-Risk List in 2015, and its continued inclusion in the 2017 and 2019 high-risk reports.[1]

Additionally, in February 2015, VHA's Task Force on Improving Effectiveness of VHA Governance produced a report with 21 recommendations for improving operational effectiveness and efficiency, including recommendations to improve operations at the VISN level.[2] The task force noted that the VISNs largely operated independently and that there was little collaboration across medical centers. Based in part on the task force's recommendations, VHA realigned the VISNs, which included decreasing the number of VISNs from 21 to 18 and reassigning some medical centers to different VISNs. In addition, the task force identified a need for VHA to focus on the composition of VISN offices in order to improve their efficiency, organizational alignment, and business outcomes.

---

[1] GAO maintains a high-risk list to focus attention on government agencies and programs that it identifies as high risk due to their greater vulnerabilities to fraud, waste, abuse, and mismanagement or the need for transformation to address economy, efficiency, or effectiveness challenges. See GAO, *High-Risk Series: An Update*, GAO-15-290 (Washington, D.C.: Feb. 11, 2015); GAO, *High-Risk Series: Progress on Many High-Risk Areas, While Substantial Effort Needed on Others*, GAO-17-317 (Washington, D.C.: Feb. 15, 2017); and GAO, High-Risk Series: Substantial Efforts Needed to Sustain Progress on High-Risk Areas, GAO-19-157SP (Washington, D.C.: Mar. 6, 2019).

[2] VHA, *Task Force on Improving Effectiveness of VHA Governance: Report to the VHA Under Secretary for Health*, (Feb. 28, 2015).

In response to one of the task force's recommendations, VHA established the VISN Staffing Task Force to consider and recommend the appropriate staffing levels and positions needed to operate the VISNs.

You asked us to conduct a review of VISNs, including VHA's oversight of VISNs. This chapter examines:

- the extent to which VHA oversees VISNs' management and oversight of medical centers; and
- how VHA oversees VISN staffing.

To examine the extent to which VHA oversees VISNs' management and oversight of medical centers, we reviewed documentation from VHA, including policies and related documents that describe VISN-level responsibilities. We also reviewed information VHA officials use to assess, monitor, compare, and manage performance across VISNs, such as VISN director performance plans. We interviewed officials from VHA's Office of the Deputy Under Secretary for Health for Operations and Management, which is responsible for VISN oversight and monitoring. We also interviewed officials from a non-generalizable sample of five VHA program offices, which develop and manage policies and programs related to: (1) homelessness, (2) mental health and suicide prevention, (3) sterile processing services, (4) community engagement, and (5) internal audits and risk assessment. We selected program offices to include those both with and without corresponding subject-matter positions at each of the 18 VISNs, to determine what, if any, oversight responsibilities these offices have over VISNs. For example, we included the VHA program office that specializes in homelessness, as each VISN must have a full-time equivalent (FTE) employee assigned to homelessness, according to VHA's standardized VISN organizational chart.[3] We interviewed officials from all 18 VISNs to obtain their perspectives on VHA's oversight. We also interviewed officials from four medical centers to obtain their perspectives on VISNs' management and oversight of their medical centers. We

[3] An FTE is a standard measure of labor that equates to one year of full-time work. See Office of Management and Budget Circular No. A-11, Sec. 85 (2018).

selected a non-generalizable sample of medical centers for variation in geographic location, VHA's categorization of medical center complexity level, urban or rural location, and VHA's 2017 star ratings.[4] We evaluated VHA's process for overseeing VISNs' management and oversight of medical centers against relevant federal standards for internal control.[5]

To examine how VHA oversees VISN staffing, we reviewed: (1) VHA policies and guidance, related to staffing, (2) related internal and external assessments of VISN staffing, and (3) organizational charts from all 18 VISNs. We also reviewed VISN staffing data from VA's core human resources processing system—HR Smart—for fiscal years 2013 through 2017. We interviewed VHA officials about how these data were collected and documented, as well as the steps taken to ensure that the data were complete. Based on this information, we determined that these data were sufficiently reliable for the purposes of our reporting objective. We also interviewed officials from VHA and the 18 VISNs about VHA's process to oversee VISN staffing. We evaluated VHA's process for overseeing VISN staffing against relevant federal standards for internal control.[6]

We conducted this performance audit from March 2018 to June 2019 in accordance with generally accepted government auditing standards. Those standards require that we plan and perform the audit to obtain sufficient, appropriate evidence to provide a reasonable basis for our findings and conclusions based on our audit objectives. We believe that the evidence obtained provides a reasonable basis for our findings and conclusions based on our audit objectives.

---

[4] VHA categorizes medical centers according to complexity level, determined on the basis of the characteristics of the patient population, clinical services offered, educational and research missions, and administrative complexity. Complexity levels range from low (level 3) to medium (level 2) to high (levels 1a, 1b, and 1c). VHA rates the overall quality of medical centers based on a star rating system of 1 (lowest) to 5 (highest) stars. VHA star ratings are based on VHA's Strategic Analytics for Improvement and Learning system, which consolidates and summarizes medical center performance information.

[5] GAO, Standards for Internal Control in the Federal Government, GAO-14-704G (Washington, D.C.: September 2014). Internal control is a process effected by an entity's oversight body, management, and other personnel that provides reasonable assurance that the objectives of an entity will be achieved.

[6] GAO-14-704G.

BACKGROUND

VHA's health care delivery system is organized regionally, around VISNs. The VISNs were established in 1995 as a part of a strategy to decentralize VA health care decisions and bring decision-making closer to the point of care. VISNs were initially designed to be the basic budgetary and planning unit of VHA. VISN directors—who each report to VHA's Deputy Under Secretary for Operations and Management—were given the autonomy and authority to develop and implement local management, administrative, and staffing arrangements when necessary to meet health care needs. Since then, the number of VISNs has decreased from the original 22 to 18, VISN boundaries have been realigned, and the staffing structure has changed to help support emerging VHA-wide health care needs. Collectively, staffing across all VISNs averaged about 1,000 FTEs each year, from fiscal years 2013 to 2018.

VISNs manage regional markets that deliver health care, social services, and support services to veterans. Each VISN is responsible for overseeing medical centers within a defined geographic area. VISNs manage the day-to-day functions of medical centers within their networks through efforts such as periodic strategic, business, and financial planning meetings. VISNs' oversight of medical centers includes the following examples:

Site Visits

VHA requires VISN officials to conduct site visits to medical centers at least twice a year. During these visits, VISN officials may review medical center operations or specific program areas and may make recommendations for improvement. According to VISN officials, some VISNs have tracking mechanisms to ensure medical centers take corrective actions, and others leave the responsibility for resolving site visit recommendations to medical centers.

Conference Calls

VISN directors and senior leadership officials told us they hold regular conference calls with medical center staff. These calls can be used to discuss current issues of interest, including process-improvement initiatives, and challenges medical centers are experiencing, among other issues.

Performance Reviews

VISN officials review a dashboard of measures to assess medical center performance.[7] The measures may include those from VHA's Strategic Analytics for Improvement and Learning (SAIL) system, which as of fiscal year 2018 included 29 performance measures (27 quality measures and 2 measures of overall efficiency and capacity) in areas such as acute care mortality, access to care, and employee satisfaction.[8] SAIL is a diagnostic tool that allows VHA to assess medical centers' performance relative to their peers, and determine year-to-year improvement based on relevant clinical data. For example, SAIL includes an online performance management tool called Symphony that tracks performance measures related to medical center access, outcomes, and productivity, and includes an early warning system to notify VISN and medical center officials of results that require action.

Best practices and regional consortiums. According to VHA, each VISN is part of a regional consortium—comprised of several VISNs in a particular geographic area—that are to share resources and best practices, conduct program reviews, and discuss common needs. Regional consortiums were formed to foster collaboration among medical centers and to enhance operations and the delivery of health care to veterans. To

---

[7] As of February 2019, VHA officials told us they are working to standardize the dashboard of measures used by VISNs.

[8] VHA created the SAIL system to measure, evaluate, and benchmark the quality, efficiency, and productivity of medical centers, and to highlight successful strategies of high performing medical centers.

accomplish these goals, the consortiums use means such as regional contracts, sharing FTEs, and joint networks for referring patients and conducting telehealth, according to VISN officials. For each regional consortium, the corresponding VISN directors serve as a board of directors to approve and guide the consortium's actions.

MAJOR FINDINGS

VHA's Oversight of VISNs Is Limited

VHA's Oversight of VISNs Relies Primarily on Individual Director Assessments

VHA officials told us they rely primarily on annual assessments of individual VISN directors' performance to assess VISN operations. Officials said they supplement these assessments with meetings with VISN leadership, including quarterly reviews of VISN performance on specific topics. These oversight activities do not provide comprehensive information on VISN-wide operations or overall performance of VISNs.

According to federal standards for internal control, management should design control activities through its policies and procedures that help it achieve its objectives, such as effective management and performance. The establishment of policies aimed at validating the propriety and integrity of both the organization and individual performance measures helps management monitor performance.[9] Additionally, the Office of Personnel Management's A Handbook for Measuring Employee Performance notes that by measuring only individual actions an organization might find that the organization as a whole has failed to meet its objectives, even if most of its employees are appraised highly.[10]

VHA officials told us that individual VISN director performance reviews, conducted annually, are VHA's primary assessment of VISN

---

[9] GAO-14-704G.

[10] U.S. Office of Personnel Management, A Handbook for Measuring Employee Performance, (Washington, D.C.: March 2017).

performance. We found that these individual assessments rely heavily on medical center information.[11] Specifically, VHA's Senior Executive Service Part V. Performance Appraisal System handbook states that VISN directors are assessed using a performance appraisal template that identifies expectations across five elements established by the Office of Personnel Management: (1) Leading Change, (2) Leading People, (3) Business Acumen, (4) Building Coalitions, and (5) Results Driven.[12] None of the five elements include performance measures or an evaluation specific to the VISN level, including its oversight of medical centers.

VHA's handbook designates a relative weight for each element used to calculate a director's rating. Sixty percent of the VISN director's performance review—assessed by the first four elements—is based on the director's individual performance. The remaining 40 percent— assessed through the Results Driven element—is based entirely on medical center performance information. SAIL results for medical centers within the VISN contribute to the Results Driven element. As noted earlier, SAIL assesses performance across a broad range of evidence-based indicators, including measures such as patient mortality, length of stay, and readmissions. Other medical center performance information, including data on access to care, comprised the remainder of the Results Driven element. VHA officials acknowledged an individual VISN directors' personal performance is not always indicative of that VISN's performance as a whole, but said the medical center performance data that inform these individual assessments is how they can best determine how well a VISN is doing leading and providing oversight to medical centers. As previously stated, it is important for an organization to have both individual and organizational-level performance measures to help monitor performance.

---

[11] We reported similar findings in a recently issued report examining VHA performance management, see GAO, Veterans Health Administration: Past Performance System Recommendations Have Not Been Implemented; GAO-19-350 (Washington, D.C.: Apr. 30, 2019).

[12] VA adopted OPM's government-wide SES performance appraisal system in fiscal year 2012 and modified it, as permitted by OPM, to address VA-unique requirements. See Department of Veterans Affairs, "Senior Executive Service, Part V. Performance Appraisal System," VA Handbook 5027/2 (Washington, D.C.: Nov. 6, 2014).

VHA officials told us they also assess VISN performance through meetings with VISN officials. For example, VHA officials told us they conduct quarterly VISN reviews that are generally about an hour in length, and involve the VISN director and the Deputy Under Secretary for Health for Operations and Management, among others. During these quarterly reviews, the VISN director uses a VHA-designated template to provide an update on the VISN's performance on specified topics. From our review of the template, we found that the quarterly reviews focus primarily on VISN-reported activities, successes and challenges.[13] They do not typically include performance measures specific to the VISN level, such as how VISNs are performing their intended roles to carry out oversight and management of medical centers. Instead, performance measures included in the quarterly review template measure medical centers' performance within a VISN, similar to some of the measures used to assess the individual performance assessment for VISN directors. For example, the quarterly template includes medical centers' SAIL metrics. In our prior work, we reported that best practices for formal assessments are to be objective and measure the results, impact, or effects of a program or policy.[14] These formal assessments can also help in determining the appropriateness of goals or the effectiveness of strategies.

VHA officials told us that they also hold periodic meetings with VISN leadership and weekly meetings with VISN directors. For example, officials from the Office of the Deputy Under Secretary for Health for Operations and Management told us they regularly meet with all VISN chief medical officers and quality management officers, as well as meet with all deputy VISN network directors. VHA officials also told us they facilitate weekly calls with all VISN directors and hold monthly meetings

---

[13] According to the template, quarterly review topics for discussion are SAIL metrics; patient surgery quality assurance metrics; any outstanding recommendations from the VA Office of Inspector General and external entities, such as GAO and the Joint Commission, a national health care accrediting body; congressional or media activities; employee engagement; and best practices.

[14] GAO, *Agencies' Strategic Plans Under GPRA: Key Questions to Facilitate Congressional Review*, GAO/GGD-10.1.16 (Washington D.C.: May 1997). GAO, *Managing for Results: Critical Issues for Improving Federal Agencies' Strategic Plans*, GAO/GGD97-180 (Washington D.C.: September 1997).

with VISN directors, as part of the National Leadership Council.[15] These calls and meetings do not include a comprehensive assessment of VISN performance, but rather serve as check-in meetings and include program office presentations. They also include discussion of any new topics of interest, or emerging or ongoing issues for VISNs or medical centers, according to VISN officials.

Although individual assessments and periodic meetings provide some useful information on how the VISN is doing in specific areas, it is also important to have a process to assess overall VISN performance in managing and overseeing medical centers. In our prior work, we reported that routine organizational assessments can provide feedback to an agency on how well day-to-day activities and programs developed to operationalize goals and objectives contribute to the achievement of those goals and objectives, such as VHA's goal to ensure effective oversight of medical centers.[16] By establishing a process for assessing the overall performance of VISNs in managing and overseeing medical centers, VHA would be better able to determine if a VISN's performance is positive, if it is functioning poorly, or if it requires remediation.

VHA Lacks a Comprehensive Policy That Defines VISN Roles and Responsibilities

VHA does not have a comprehensive policy that defines VISNs' roles and responsibilities to manage and oversee medical centers. This is contrary to federal standards for internal control, which call for management to assign responsibilities and hold individuals accountable, and for management to consider how components interact within the whole organization in order to fulfill responsibilities and meet operating objectives.[17] VHA requires the use of policy to assign responsibilities for

[15] The National Leadership Council is the Under Secretary for Health's governance structure for all VHA policies, plans, and procedures. It is comprised of VHA and VISN officials in leadership positions.

[16] GAO/GGD-97-180 and GAO/GGD-10.1.16.

[17] GAO-14-704G.

executing a course of action to individuals or groups.[18] VHA and VISN officials told us that although they do not have a comprehensive policy that clearly documents VISN roles and responsibilities, they have several documents they believe help VISNs understand their roles and responsibilities. These documents include program office policies, VISN directors' job descriptions, and a newly developed Network Director Playbook. However, our review of these documents found that they lack broader VISN-level responsibilities, as described below.

Program Office Policies

In our review of program office policies, we found high-level outlines of VISN director responsibilities for implementing specific policies or programs, but these outlines did not detail broader VISN-level responsibilities, such as what the VISN is expected to do to manage and oversee medical centers. For example, a VHA directive on homelessness states that the VISN director is responsible for ensuring veterans have timely access to VHA homeless programs and services at medical centers, as well as ensuring quality care for veterans. However, this directive does not discuss other VISN responsibilities outside of the director or for areas outside of the specific program area. Additionally, although VISN director responsibilities are outlined in policies, VHA officials told us that program offices do not have direct oversight responsibilities of VISNs. As previously noted, VISN directors report to the Deputy Under Secretary for Health for Operations and Management.

VISN Director Job Descriptions

Job descriptions state that VISN directors are expected to provide leadership and management skills in various areas, such as strategic planning, quality assessments, and human resources, as well as establish operational, financial and strategic plans for the VISN. The VISN director

---

[18] Department of Veterans Affairs, Veterans Health Administration, VHA Directive 6330 (4): Controlled National Policy/Directives Management System, (Washington D.C.: June 24, 2016). (Amended June 29, 2018.)

job descriptions are tied to an individual position and do not clearly describe what the VISN as a whole is responsible for accomplishing.

Network Director Playbook

VISN officials told us that they developed a Network Director Playbook to reduce variation in VISNs. The playbook describes the responsibilities of VISN directors as (1) managing regional markets that deliver health care, social services, and support services to veterans, and (2) providing administrative and clinical oversight of medical centers. The playbook also highlights seven high-level topic areas pertaining to VISN-level roles, but it does not include additional detail on what is expected of the VISN, nor does it provide goals for what is to be achieved in these areas.[19] The remainder of the playbook provides a resource guide and primer for VISN directors on various topics. For example, the playbook includes resource chapters on administrative investigations, the communication process, governance, and other topics related to VISNs' management and oversight of medical centers. VHA officials noted that the playbook is guidance rather than policy. Officials we interviewed from four VISNs agreed, stating that the playbook was meant to serve as a guide when needed, but is not required to be followed. One VISN director told us that he does not use the playbook because he views it as a guide only for new VISN directors.

The lack of a comprehensive policy defining VISN-level roles and responsibilities for managing and overseeing medical centers makes it difficult for VHA to develop an effective oversight process that ensures adequate monitoring of VISN activities and a way to address poorly performing VISNs. The Task Force on Improving Effectiveness of VHA Governance 2015 report included a recommendation for VHA to articulate the work and roles and responsibilities of the VISNs, and provided a

---

[19] The seven areas outlined in the playbook are: (1) drive strategic investment, (2) oversee clinical and financial management, (3) translate national policy and strategy into action, (4) identify and mitigate risk, (5) ensure compliance with external inspections, (6) oversee effective performance, and (7) drive market assessments.

framework and suggested roles.[20] In response to this recommendation, VHA officials told us they have taken several steps, which include the standardization of the VISN governance process and expanding the VISNs' role in key operational elements, such as contracting and information technology. Additionally, in 2018, VHA conducted a review of the VISN structure to inform a VISN redesign process.[21] The resulting December 2018 Veterans Integrated Services Networks (VISN) Redesign Report also noted the lack of clearly defined roles and responsibilities at the VISN level. Clearly defined roles and responsibilities would better position VHA to develop an oversight process to effectively assess overall VISN performance in managing and overseeing medical centers.

VHA Has Standardized VISN Staffing Levels and Positions, but Does Not Ensure VISNs Adhere to Them

VHA has standardized staffing levels and positions for VISN staffing, but we found that VHA does not fully monitor VISNs' adherence to them. VHA uses a standardized VISN organizational chart to document these staffing levels and positions. (See appendix I for VHA's standardized VISN organizational chart.) The standardized chart was developed by the VISN Staffing Task Force, which VHA established in 2015 to recommend the appropriate staffing levels and mix of positions to effectively operate VISNs and to standardize key functions.[22] The Deputy Under Secretary for Health for Operations and Management approved the standardized organizational chart in July 2016. VHA officials told us they expect VISNs to adhere to it.

---

[20] Department of Veterans Affairs, Veterans Health Administration, Task Force on Improving Effectiveness of VHA Governance: Report to the VHA Under Secretary for Health, (Washington, D.C.: Feb. 28, 2015).

[21] This report also included recommendations related to VISN governance, leadership, processes, and performance management. Department of Veterans Affairs, Veterans Integrated Services Networks (VISN) Redesign Report, (Washington, D.C.: December 2018).

[22] Members of the task force included VISN directors, the Deputy Under Secretary for Health for Clinical Operations, a patient care services officer, and a VISN chief medical officer.

According to VHA's standardized VISN staffing levels, each VISN is allowed between 63 and 66 FTE staff based on the VISN's complexity, veteran demographics, and the health of the veteran population served by its medical centers. These VISN staff are responsible for carrying out the functions of the VISN for overseeing and managing medical centers, including implementing national policies and programs, managing internal and external relationships, and sharing best practices. The standardized VISN organizational chart also contains 28 key positions (each representing one FTE unless otherwise noted) that should be in place at every VISN, including a chief medical officer, mental health lead, and patient safety officer. Additionally, the organizational chart contains a specific staffing composition for each VISN: 44 base positions, six administrative positions, 12 clinical or administrative analytical positions, and up to four adjustment positions based on the size of the VISN.[23]

VHA officials told us that to oversee staffing, they compared VISNs' organizational charts to VHA's standardized organizational chart. Specifically, on June 14, 2018, the Office of the Deputy Under Secretary for Health emailed all VISN directors to request that they align their individual staffing levels and positions to the standardized chart, document any changes as a result of the alignment on their individual VISN organizational charts, and submit them by June 22, 2018, to the Deputy Under Secretary for Health for Operations and Management for review and approval. Apart from this one-time review and approval process, VHA officials told us they do not have an oversight process to review VISN organizational charts on a regular basis.[24]

VHA officials told us the process VHA used to review VISNs' organizational charts involved checking that VISNs' reported total FTEs were within the allotted allowance and adhered to the staffing composition.

---

23 Base positions are those linked to specific VISN functions recommended by VHA's Task Force on Improving Effectiveness of VHA Governance. For example, the Capital Asset Manager base position is linked to functions that include operationalizing national policies and programs and coordinating communications with VHA. Adjustment positions are those left to the discretion of the VISN for its individual needs.

24 VHA officials told us that they also review VISNs' organizational charts on an ad hoc basis, such as when VISNs want to make changes to their organizational charts. In these instances, organizational charts are resubmitted for approval.

As of February 2019, VHA had approved the organizational charts for 15 of 18 VISNs based on the standardized VISN organizational chart. According to officials, the remaining three VISNs had either not submitted a chart for review or not had their chart approved.

VHA's review and approval process did not ensure that VISN organizational charts always included the 28 key positions. In our analysis comparing the 15 approved VISN organizational charts to the standardized chart, we found one to five key positions were not listed on the organizational charts of six of the 15 VISNs with approved organizational charts[25] For example, one VISN was missing both the primary care and geriatrics and extended care positions on its organizational chart. VISN officials provided various reasons for the positions not being listed on the organizational charts. For example, VISN officials said that in several instances the position did not appear on the chart because these responsibilities were being performed as a collateral duty—taken on in addition to normal duties—for a staff person at the VISN or at one of the medical centers in the VISN.[26]

VHA officials told us there is some limited flexibility in the standardized VISN organizational chart. However, they also said that they have not documented the criteria for approving VISNs' organizational charts that do not adhere to the standardized chart, nor have they documented approvals that have allowed for flexibility.

VHA officials told us they also did not confirm that VISNs staffed the key positions listed in their organizational charts. In our analysis of VISNs' organizational charts, we compared positions listed on each chart with VISN data about staff employed at each of the VISNs as documented in VA's HR Smart system.[27]

---

[25] One VISN was missing five key positions, a second VISN was missing three, a third VISN was missing two, and three VISNs were missing one.

[26] Officials from another VISN told us the position existed at the VISN, but had not been included on the organizational chart.

[27] HR Smart includes data on positions encumbered with current VA employees and vacant positions.

We found that most position titles in HR Smart did not match position titles in the organizational charts, and VHA officials told us that no position-title crosswalk exists. The lack of a crosswalk limits VHA's ability to monitor VISN staffing on an ongoing basis and ensure that the VISNs are staffed consistently with the standardized organizational chart. VHA officials told us that they expect VISNs to accurately report their staffing compositions via their organizational charts, and acknowledge they do not assess the extent to which this occurs.

VHA's current monitoring of VISN staffing is inconsistent with federal standards for internal control, which state that management should establish and operate monitoring activities and evaluate the results.[28] Establishing a process to routinely oversee staffing would help VHA ensure VISNs staff the positions it has determined necessary for effective operations and would provide VHA leadership with greater assurance that key positions—as determined by the standardized VISN organizational chart—are filled at the VISNs.

CONCLUSION

Given VISNs' responsibilities for managing and overseeing VA medical centers, it is important that VHA have a robust process for ensuring that VISNs function as intended. Although VHA gathers information on VISN director performance, and on specific aspects of VISN operations, establishing a process for assessing the overall performance of VISNs would enable VHA to better determine how VISNs are performing. Furthermore, a comprehensive policy clearly defining VISN roles and responsibilities would better enable VHA to develop an effective oversight process to ensure adequate monitoring of VISN activities and a way to address poorly performing VISNs.

---

[28] GAO-14-704G.

Additionally, creating a process to oversee VISN staffing would help VHA ensure VISNs adhere to established staffing levels and positions. The lack of clearly defined roles and responsibilities leaves VHA challenged to determine whether its expectations of VISN staffing levels- and positions are appropriate. By establishing a process for routine oversight of staffing, VHA would have greater assurances that VISNs have the staff in place that VHA has determined are needed to effectively operate VISNs. A lack of appropriate staffing could hinder VISNs' ability to oversee the care that VA medical centers provide to veterans.

Agency Comments and Our Evaluation

We provided VA with a draft of this chapter for review and comment. VA provided written comments, which are reprinted in appendix II. In its comments, VA noted that VHA's plan to modernize its governance structure, clinical services, human resources, and organizational structure, in addition to other efforts, will address all three of our recommendations.

VA concurred with two of our recommendations—for VHA to develop a process to assess the overall performance of VISNs and to establish a process to routinely oversee VISN staffing—and provided information on how implementation of its modernization efforts will address them, with targeted completion dates of November 2019 and March 2020, respectively. VA concurred in principle with our recommendation for VHA to establish a comprehensive policy clearly defining VISN roles and responsibilities for managing and overseeing medical centers. In its comments, VA noted that providing written guidance outlining oversight roles and responsibilities for all levels of the organization is part of its planned modernization efforts and that it expects this guidance will define VISN roles and responsibilities. VA provided a target completion date for the recommendation of November 2019.

VA added that this guidance may take various forms, including governance principles, standard operating procedures, and decision authorities.

Although these guidance documents may clarify VISN roles and responsibilities, they do not denote a comprehensive policy, and as we described in our report VHA requires the use of policy to assign responsibilities for executing a course of action to individuals or groups. Therefore, we maintain that VA should establish a comprehensive policy that clearly defines VISN roles and responsibilities for managing and overseeing medical centers.

We are sending copies of this chapter to the appropriate congressional committees, the Secretary of Veterans Affairs, and other interested parties.

Debra A. Draper
Director, Health Care

List of Congressional Addressees

The Honorable Julia Brownley
Chair

The Honorable Neal Dunn
Ranking Member
Subcommittee on Health
Committee on Veterans' Affairs
House of Representatives

The Honorable Peter A. DeFazio
House of Representatives

The Honorable Ann McLane Kuster
House of Representatives

The Honorable Brad Wenstrup
House of Representatives

APPENDIX I: VETERANS HEALTH ADMINISTRATION (VHA) STANDARDIZED VETERANS INTEGRATED SERVICE NETWORK ORGANIZATIONAL CHART, AS OF JULY 2016

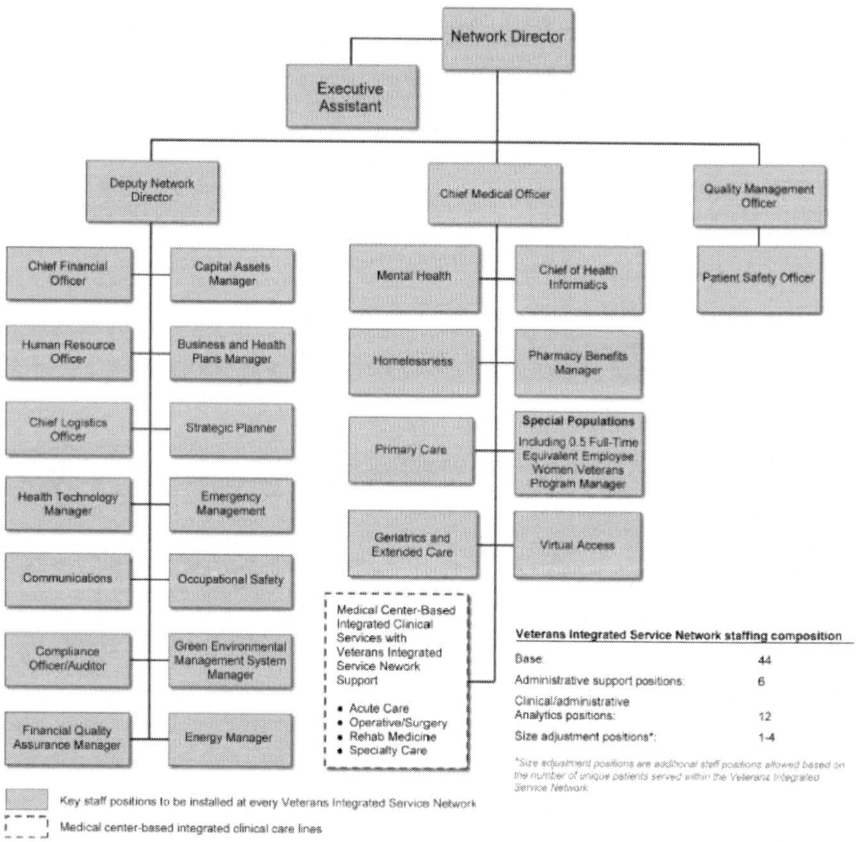

Source: Veteran's Health Administration.| GAO-19-482.

Appendix II: Comments from the Department of Veterans Affairs

THE SECRETARY OF VETERANS AFFAIRS
WASHINGTON

May 22, 2019

Ms. Debra A. Draper
Director
Health Care
U.S. Government Accountability Office
441 G Street, NW
Washington, DC 20548

Dear Ms. Draper:

The Department of Veterans Affairs (VA) has reviewed the Government Accountability Office (GAO) draft report: *VETERANS HEALTH ADMINISTRATION: Regional Networks Need Improved Oversight and Clearly Defined Roles and Responsibilities* (GAO-19-462). The enclosure includes our general comments and sets forth the actions to be taken to address the draft report recommendations.

VA appreciates the opportunity to comment on your draft report.

Sincerely,

Robert L. Wilkie

Department of Veterans Affairs (VA) Comments to
Government Accountability Office (GAO) Draft Report
VETERANS HEALTH ADMINISTRATION: Regional Networks Need Improved Oversight and Clearly Defined Roles and Responsibilities
(GAO-19-462)

General Comments:

The Veterans Health Administration (VHA) appreciates the U.S. Government Accountability Office (GAO) review of our regional networks – known as Veterans Integrated Service Networks (VISN). GAO's findings support VHA's plan for modernization to our governance structure, clinical service lines, shared services, and streamlining headquarters. We are confident that full implementation of our modernization efforts will resolve GAO's concerns. We are grateful for GAO's insight and recommendations for improved oversight of the current VISN structure and function.

We define our vision for a modernized VHA simply as: Consistent delivery of excellent quality care and customer service for every patient, every time. VHA's Plan for Modernization focuses on both the infrastructure and the cultural changes necessary to create high reliability for the Veterans we serve every single day. We are committed to new investments that will help all employees – in care delivery sites, VISNs, and Central Office (CO) – work together to create our modernized VHA.

The following four lanes of effort, taken together, significantly impact the structure, function, and oversight of regional networks.

Revise Governance Processes and Align Decision Rights. VHA is simplifying its governance structure to empower employees to make decisions at all levels – supported by agreed-upon roles, responsibilities, accountability, and decision-making authority. This year, the current governing body is being replaced by a Board of Governors; membership includes leaders from the VISNs and headquarters. The transformed governance system follows established decision criteria outlining the types of decisions that are made at each level of governance, including VISN and facility level decisions. Using these decision criteria, leaders will more clearly understand their level of authority, roles, and responsibilities.

Reduce Unwarranted Variation Across Integrated Clinical and Operational Service Lines. VHA is aligning clinical services into six clinical service lines: mental health, primary care, surgery, diagnostics, rehabilitation, extended care, and specialty care. Clinical services are to have mirrored structures, roles, and responsibilities at health care facilities, VISNs, and CO. Facility level clinical services and programs align to their respective VISN structure, and the VISN structure is to be mirrored at CO. Common clinical and operational structure throughout the organization drives a consistent Veteran and employee experience, enables rapid flow of information and best practices vertically and horizontally throughout the organization, supports the development of VHA as a learning organization and a high-reliability organization. Vertically aligned clinical service lines in concert with establishing shared services impact VISN staffing and function.

Develop Responsive Shared Services. During Fiscal Years 2019 and 2020, modernization efforts consolidate human resource functions from more than 140 local facilities into shared services managed at the regional level by 18 VISNs. Expected results include: streamlined human resource services; standardized processes; and an enabled enterprise that can recruit and hire needed staff in an effective and efficient manner. Developing responsive shared human resources services managed at the VISN level will enhance VHA's ability to fill vacant and essential health care positions more rapidly and provide high-quality human resource services to VHA employees. Consolidation of human resource services to the VISN level significantly impacts VISN staffing and function.

Streamline VHA Central Office. VHA's organizational structure is complex, with many offices that have evident functional overlaps. Inefficiencies created by CO's structure overburdens VISNs and facilities and contributes to confusion about roles, responsibilities and authorities. VHA is flattening the organizational structure by consolidating program offices with similar functions. The future state organizational design aligns CO, VISN, and facility structures to support and facilitate vertical and horizontal integration. Improved coordination with community health providers will create the largest, highest-functioning integrated health system in the United States. Additionally, a more efficient, more effective, and more accountable VHA should restore Veterans trust in VHA to meet their health care needs – every time.

VHA's plan for Modernization builds an infrastructure that allows VHA to become an integrated, high-performing, high reliability organization. In addition to the four lanes of effort described above, the total ten lanes of modernization efforts drive both short- and long-term improvements everywhere VHA delivers care to Veterans. The ten lanes of modernization efforts for VHA are:

- Commit to Zero Harm;
- VA Maintaining Internal Systems and Strengthening Integrated Outside Networks (MISSION) Act: Improve Access to Care;
- Engaging Veterans in Lifelong Health, Well-Being, and Resilience;
- Reduce Unwarranted Variation Across Integrated Clinical and Operational Service Lines;
- Streamline VHA Central Office;

- Revise Governance processes and Align Decision Rights;
- Develop Responsive Shared Services;
- Modernize Electronic Health Records;
- Transform Financial Management System; and
- Transform Supply Chain.

Recommendation 1: **The Under Secretary for Health should develop a process to assess the overall performance of VISNs in managing and overseeing medical centers.**

VA Comment: Concur. The Government Accountability Office (GAO) findings from this review soundly support Veterans Health Administration's (VHA) plan for modernizing our governance structure. VHA is simplifying its governance structure to empower employees to make decisions at the appropriate level, moving decision authority closer to the point of care – supported by agreed-upon roles, responsibilities, accountability, and decision-making authority. Later this year, the current governing body is being replaced by a Board of Governors formed by Veterans Integrated Services Network (VISN) and national program office leaders. The transformed governance system follows established decision criteria outlining the types of decisions that are made at each level of governance, especially VISN and facility-level decisions. Using decision criteria, leaders will more clearly understand their level of authority, roles, and responsibilities. We are confident that full implementation of modernization efforts will resolve GAO's concerns with respect to processes for assessing VISN performance in managing and overseeing medical centers. Target Completion Date: November 2019

Recommendation 2: **The Under Secretary for Health should establish a comprehensive policy that clearly defines VISN roles and responsibilities for managing and overseeing medical centers.**

VA Comment: Concur in principle. We are grateful for GAO's insight and attention to the need for clear definitions for VISN roles and responsibilities with respect to managing and overseeing medical centers. Written guidance outlining oversight roles and responsibilities for Central Office governance bodies, VISN, and facility Directors are part of VISNs modernization efforts to revise governance processes and align decision rights. We expect written guidance will clearly define VISN roles and responsibilities. This guidance may take many forms, such as: governance principles, guidance for good governance, decision authorities, standard operating procedures, oversight responsibilities, etc. We are confident that full implementation of modernization efforts will resolve GAO's concerns with respect to clarification of VISN oversight roles and responsibilities. Target Completion Date: November 2019

Recommendation 3: **The Under Secretary for Health should establish process to routinely oversee VISN staffing, to include ensuring VISNs are consistent with VHA's standardized VISN staffing levels and positions and documenting the**

rationale for approving staffing that does not adhere to VHA's standardized approach.

VA Comment: Concur. VHA concurs that the oversight of VISNs can be enhanced to ensure sound position management. Networks do not need to be identical, due to variations in size, types of facilities, and challenges, but all need to ensure appropriate oversight of all activities. As VISN organizational charts are revised based on modernization plans, VHA will be instituting a review of the accuracy and consistency of VISN staffing by VHA's Office of Workforce Management and Consulting prior to approval by the Deputy Undersecretary for Health for Operations and Management. Target Completion Date: March 2020

In: Key Government Reports. Volume 26 ISBN: 978-1-53616-568-5
Editor: Ernest Clark

Chapter 5

VA Real Property: Improvements in Facility Planning Needed to Ensure VA Meets Changes in Veterans' Needs and Expectations*

United States Government Accountability Office

Abbreviations

SCIP	Strategic Capital Investment Planning
VA	Department of Veterans Affairs
VAMC	VA medical center
VetPop2016	Veteran Population Projection Model 2016
VHA	Veterans Health Administration

* This is an edited, reformatted and augmented version of United States Government Accountability Office; Report to Congressional Requesters, Accessible Version, Publication No. GAO-19-440, dated June 13, 2019.

VISN	Veterans Integrated Service Network
VSO	veterans service organization

WHY GAO DID THIS STUDY

VA provides for care to over 9-million veterans in its health care system, including 172 VAMCs. As veterans' demographics shift, such as by age or gender, their needs for health care and their expectations for how they receive that care may also change. Along with the VA MISSION Act of 2018, which requires VA to assess its facilities for realignment and modernization, these changes could have implications for VA's capital-planning efforts.

GAO was asked to review how VA incorporates veterans' changing needs and expectations into facility planning. This chapter examines: (1) VA's efforts to assess trends in veterans' future needs and expectations; (2) VA's efforts to help VAMCs address these changes through facility planning; and (3) how VAMCs use VA's process for identifying facilities' future space needs.

GAO surveyed all VAMCs, visited nine VAMCs, reviewed VA's planning documents and data, and interviewed officials from VA and veterans service organizations. GAO's survey response rate was 99 percent.

WHAT GAO RECOMMENDS

GAO recommends VA: (1) assess changes in veterans' expectations; (2) instruct facility planners on how to incorporate veterans' changing needs and expectations; (3) clarify foundational health services implementation; and (4) assess concerns with the SCIP process and make needed adjustments. VA agreed with GAO's recommendations.

What GAO Found

The Department of Veterans Affairs (VA) analyzes demographic trends to assess veterans' future health-care needs, such as the need for more long-term care or women's health care services. VA does not, however, systematically collect data concerning whether demographic groups differ in their expectations for how they will receive care, such as whether some groups expect different levels of privacy. VA officials said they gauge expectations by surveying veterans and talking to veterans service organizations. GAO's review, however, found the amount of information VA collected through these methods is limited. Without robust data about veterans' expectations and assessing how changes would affect facilities' space needs, VA cannot readily anticipate and adapt to meet veterans' changing expectations—a goal in its *FY 2018–2024 Strategic Plan*.

In addition to identifying meeting veterans' changing needs and expectations as a national strategic goal, VA defined a national set of VA-delivered core medical services called "foundational health services" to, in part, meet veterans' expectations of consistent care offerings across VA medical centers (VAMC) and also to focus VA's resources on its highest priority services. However, based on GAO's survey of VAMCs and discussions with selected facility-planning officials, GAO found that VA did not clearly instruct VAMCs in how to apply VA's strategic goal or foundational health services to facility planning. Accordingly, more than three quarters of VAMC facility-planning officials responding to GAO's survey indicated additional instruction from VA for the strategic goal and foundational health services would be useful. Without providing clear instruction, VA increases its risk that its strategic goal and foundational health services are not meeting their objective to incorporate veterans' changing needs and expectations.

Most facility-planning officials had concerns with using estimated space needs derived from VA's Strategic Capital Investment Planning (SCIP) process, which converts estimated needs for veterans' health care into future space needs for the VAMCs. Specifically, the officials (1) did not understand how the SCIP process converts health care needs into physical space and (2) questioned how accurately the space estimates reflected the future health-care needs for local facilities. For example, 72 percent of facility-planning officials responding to GAO's survey reported that at least one of SCIP's 12 space category estimates was "generally inaccurate" at reflecting projected space needs for their facility. As a result, instead of relying on SCIP's space estimates as a starting point to incorporate veterans' changing needs into facility planning, VAMC facility planners told GAO that they may instead use locally identified health care needs and priorities to determine space needs. Without a process for VA to understand and address concerns about the SCIP process, VAMCs may spend time and resources on capital projects that do not necessarily meet veterans' future needs as VA intended. This approach may therefore impede VA's ability to respond to veterans needs as this population changes.

June 13, 2019

The Honorable Johnny Isakson
Chairman

The Honorable Jon Tester
Ranking Member
Committee on Veterans' Affairs
United States Senate

The Honorable Jerry Moran
United States Senate

The Department of Veterans Affairs (VA) operates one of the largest health care systems in the country. VA provides for care at 172 VA medical centers (VAMC) and 1,069 outpatient sites to over 9 million veterans enrolled in the VA health care program.[1] VA provides medical

---

[1] Outpatient facilities include community-based outpatient clinics and health care centers. Community-based outpatient clinics are located in areas surrounding VA medical centers and

services to various veteran populations, including an aging veteran population and a growing number of younger veterans returning from military operations in Afghanistan and Iraq. These and other demographic shifts in the population served by VA are expected to drive changes in veterans' needs for care and in their expectations for how their care will be delivered. These changes will have implications for VA's capital-planning efforts that are primarily undertaken by the VAMCs, and can take 4–9 years to complete.[2] This is in addition to recent requirements under the VA MISSION Act of 2018 for VA to establish criteria for assessing and making recommendations on the modernization and realignment of VA facilities.[3]

The need for VA to align its capital planning to veterans' changing demographics, and the resultant changes in their needs and expectations, is related to two high-risk areas GAO identified. One is veterans' health care, which has had systemic and persistent problems with timeliness, cost-effectiveness, quality, and safety of the care that veterans receive.[4] The

provide primary care and some specialty care services that do not require a hospital stay. Health care centers, including ambulatory care centers, are large multi-specialty outpatient clinics that provide surgical services in addition to other health care services.

[2] In 2013, GAO reported on four major construction projects for VAMCs, noting that the estimated time frames for completion were between 4 and 9 years without any delays. According to VA, the estimated completion dates are from the initial budget prospectus, which assumed receipt of all requested construction funding within 1 to 2 years after the budget submission. See GAO, *VA Construction: Additional Actions Needed to Decrease Delays and Lower Costs of Major Medical-Facility Projects*, GAO-13-302 (Washington, D.C.: Apr. 4, 2013).

[3] The criteria shall include the preferences of veterans regarding health care furnished by VA. An independent commission, the Asset and Infrastructure Review Commission, will review and analyze VA's recommendations and report its findings and conclusions to the President. VA MISSION Act of 2018. Pub. L. No. 115-182, tit. II, § 203, 132 Stat. 1393, _ (2018).

[4] GAO, *High-Risk Series: An Update,* GAO-15-290 (Washington, D.C.: February 2015). GAO maintains a high-risk program to focus attention on government operations that it identifies as high risk due to their greater vulnerabilities to fraud, waste, abuse, and mismanagement or the need for transformation to address economy, efficiency, or effectiveness challenges. See, for example, GAO, *VA Health Care: Actions Needed to Improve Oversight of Community-Based Outpatient Clinics,* GAO-18-375 (Washington, D.C.: Apr. 12, 2018) and GAO, *VA Health Care: Improved Policies and Oversight Needed for Reviewing and Reporting Providers for Quality and Safety Concerns,* GAO-18-63 (Washington, D.C.: Nov. 15 2017). See also, for example, Department of Veterans Affairs, Office of Inspector General, *Veterans Health Administration, Comprehensive Healthcare Inspection Program Review of the Washington DC VA Medical Center,* Report No. 17- 01757-50 (Washington, D.C.: Jan. 28, 2019) and VA, *Veterans Health Administration, Patient and Radiation Safety*

other is federal real property management, which includes VA's management of its real property assets—including the effective disposal of excess and underutilized VA property.[5]

You asked us to review issues related to how VA incorporates changing veterans' needs and expectations into facility planning. In this chapter, we examine:

1. The extent to which VA assesses trends in veterans' future needs and expectations.
2. VA's efforts to help VAMCs address veterans' changing needs and expectations in their facility planning.
3. How VAMCs use VA's planning process for identifying future need for space in VA's facilities to address veterans' changing needs in facility planning.

To address these objectives, we reviewed relevant laws, regulations, policies, and VA's planning documents and interviewed officials from VA and a broad range of national veterans' service organizations (VSO). To obtain local perspectives on the objectives, we surveyed those officials who are responsible for planning and making facility-planning decisions (hereafter referred to as "facility-planning officials") at all VAMCs across the country. The survey addressed VA's efforts to assess trends in veterans' needs and expectations and incorporate the information in facility planning, and VA's Strategic Capital Investment Planning (SCIP) process. We administered our web-based survey between November 2018 and January 2019 and received a 99 percent response rate.[6] See appendix I for more information about our methodology and appendix II for the survey

---

Concerns at the John D. Dingell VA Medical Center, Detroit, Michigan, Report No. 18-02210-19 (Washington, D.C.: Nov. 27, 2018).

[5] See GAO, *High-Risk Series: Federal Real Property,* GAO-03-122 (Washington, D.C.: January 2003) and GAO, *VA Real Property: Clear Procedures and Improved Data Collection Could Facilitate Property Disposals*, GAO-19-148 (Washington, D.C.: Jan. 9, 2019).

[6] We received responses from 137 of the 139 facility-planning officials, representing 159 of the 162 VAMCs. Although there are 172 VAMCs, a VA official who oversees SCIP told us that VA combines several VAMC's SCIP space gap estimates as part of the SCIP planning process. As a result, VA attributes SCIP data to 162 VAMCs.

questions and summarized responses. For more detailed information to supplement the survey, we visited a nongeneralizable sample of nine VAMCs located in four Veterans Integrated Service Networks (VISN) in August 2018 and September 2018.[7] We chose the nine VAMCs because they had relatively high future-space needs based on fiscal year 2019 data from VA's SCIP process and geographic proximity to each other. We interviewed facility-planning officials at both the VISN and VAMC levels to discuss facility-planning resources, tools, and policies, and reviewed relevant documentation provided by these officials. Even though we visited nine VAMCs, we only met with eight groups of facility-planning officials because two of the VAMCs share a common set of facility-planning officials.[8]

To determine the extent to which VA assesses trends in veterans' needs and expectations, we reviewed documentation of the Enrollee Health Care Projection Model—a VA model for estimating the amount of resources VA needs to meet the expected demand for most of the health care services it provides—and interviewed officials at VHA's Office of Policy and Planning who oversee the model to discuss projections of veterans' populations and trends.[9] We reviewed the model's documentation related to its purpose and structure and interviewed relevant officials, and determined that the data from the Enrollee Health Care Projection Model were sufficiently reliable for our audit objectives.[10] We also coordinated with VHA officials and relevant VAMC officials to

---

[7] VA organizes its system of care into regional networks called VISNs. Each VISN is responsible for managing and overseeing VA medical centers within a defined geographic area. We met with the planning officials at VISN 5 (District of Columbia, Maryland, Pennsylvania, Virginia, and West Virginia), VISN 6 (North Carolina and Virginia), VISN 8 (Florida, Georgia, Puerto Rico, and the U.S. Virgin Islands), and VISN 17 (Texas).

[8] Two of the VAMCs we visited, the Baltimore VAMC and Perry Point VAMC, are part of the VA Maryland Healthcare System and, as a result, have the same facility-planning officials. In many areas of the country, several medical centers and clinics may work together to offer services to area veterans as a health care system. According to VA, by sharing services between or among medical centers, the aim is for VHA to provide veterans easier access to advanced medical care closer to their homes.

[9] The Enrollee Health Care Projection Model was developed in 1998 by VA and its consultant. It helps supports the development of VA's budget estimates for health care and informs strategic and capital planning.

[10] A review of the underlying assumptions of the Enrollee Health Care Projection Model and the accuracy of model projections was outside the scope of this review.

identify 127 surveys that VA had been administering. In reviewing survey titles and coordinating with relevant survey points of contact, we narrowed down the 127 surveys to a list of 14 surveys by identifying those that could (1) potentially help VA understand veterans' needs and/or expectations in facility planning and (2) be attributed to different veteran population demographics (e.g., gender, age, race, etc.). We then reviewed these 14 survey instruments to determine the extent to which they included measures that specifically asked about veterans' expectations. Further, we compared VA's efforts to assess trends in veterans' needs and expectations to federal standards for internal control for use of quality information and relevant control activities.[11]

To identify what national efforts VA has initiated to help VAMCs address veterans' changing needs and expectations in facility planning, we reviewed VA documents and interviewed VA officials. To obtain local perspectives on these efforts, we spoke with the facility-planning officials at each of the VISNs and VAMCs from our nine site visits and included questions about VA's instructions to VAMCs to implement these efforts in our national survey of facility planners. Further, we compared VA's national efforts to federal standards for internal control for communicating internally and relevant control activities.[12]

To determine how facility-planning officials at VAMCs use VA's process for identifying future facilities' space needs to address veterans' changing needs and expectations in their facility planning, we used information collected from our survey and interviews with facility-planning officials at VISNs and VAMCs. We also analyzed variation in SCIP's 10-year estimates of facilities' space needs for all VAMCs across 4 years of SCIP data (SCIP fiscal years 2017, 2018, 2019, and 2020 estimates).[13] To assess the reliability of these data, we

---

[11] GAO, *Standards for Internal Control in the Federal Government*, GAO-14-704G (Washington, D.C.: September 2014).

[12] See GAO-14-704G.

[13] A given fiscal year's SCIP data are based on information collected 4 years prior. For example, SCIP data for fiscal year 2020 are based on information collected in fiscal year 2016, while SCIP data for fiscal year 2019 are based on information collected in fiscal year 2015.

- performed electronic testing of relevant data elements,
- reviewed existing information about the data and the system that produced them, and
- interviewed agency officials knowledgeable about the data.

We determined that these data were sufficiently reliable for presenting the estimates across the 4-year period. Further, we compared how VAMCs are using VA space estimates in their facility planning to federal standards for internal control for use of quality information and relevant control activities.[14]

We conducted this performance audit from April 2018 to June 2019 in accordance with generally accepted government auditing standards. Those standards require that we plan and perform the audit to obtain sufficient, appropriate evidence to provide a reasonable basis for our findings and conclusions based on our audit objectives. We believe that the evidence obtained provides a reasonable basis for our findings and conclusions based on our audit objectives. Further details on our scope and methodology can be found in appendix I.

BACKGROUND

VA's Organization

VA's mission is to serve America's veterans, and one of the ways it accomplishes this mission is by providing veterans with medical services. In general, veterans must enroll in VA health care to receive VA's medical benefits package—a set of services that includes a full range of hospital and outpatient services, prescription drugs, and long-term care services. In addition to care provided at VA medical facilities, veterans may also obtain services from non-VA providers in the community—known as community care—through one of several community-care programs aimed at helping

[14] See GAO-14-704G.

ensure veterans receive timely and accessible care. The VA MISSION Act of 2018 has introduced new eligibility criteria that could lead veterans to make increased use of community care, which may in turn affect veteran's future needs and expectations.[15]

VHA is responsible for overseeing the delivery of care to enrolled veterans, as well as overseeing the health care professionals and support staff who deliver that care. VHA is also responsible for managing all VA medical facilities across 18 regional networks, known as VISNs, which are structured to manage and allocate resources to VA's health care facilities. Each VISN is also responsible for the coordination and oversight of all administrative and clinical activities within its specified region of the country.

VA's Projection Models and Health Care Planning

VA's FY 2018–2024 Strategic Plan calls for VA to continuously adapt its benefits and health care offerings to meet veterans' changing needs and expectations.[16] VA expects that veterans' health care needs and expectations will change due to changes in veteran demographics, and VA uses several models to estimate these demographic changes. One of these models is VetPop2016, which estimates the number and key demographic characteristics of the total veterans' population—such as age, gender, period of service, and race/ethnicity—over the next 30 years. Another model that VA uses to estimate future veteran demographic characteristics is the Enrollee Health Care Projection Model—which VA told us was updated almost annually. Based on a set of assumptions, including future enrollee demographics, this model estimates the number of enrolled veterans, as well as the extent to which they will rely on VA health care and utilize services over the next 20 years.[17] As part of its health care

---

[15] VA MISSION Act of 2018. Pub. L. No. 115-182, tit. I, 132 Stat. 1393 (2018).

[16] See Department of Veterans Affairs, *FY 2018–2024 Strategic Plan* (February 2018).

[17] In determining estimates using the Enrollee Health Care Projection Model, VA uses different sets of assumptions for future years, called "scenarios," to model the impact of changes such as new policies, regulations, or legislation. For example, one scenario might assume

planning, the Enrollee Health Care Projection Model makes a number of adjustments to projections for VA's health care services to account for the characteristics of VA health care and enrolled veterans. For example, the Enrollee Health Care Projection Model includes adjustments to account for enrollees' reliance on VA health care; in other words, the extent to which enrolled veterans choose to access health care services through VA instead of obtaining services through the community. Additionally, the Enrollee Health Care Projection Model includes adjustments to incorporate the age, gender, priority level, and geographic location of enrolled veterans. The information obtained from VA's health care planning is relevant to VA's capital planning.

Capital Planning at the VA Level

VA's main mechanism for identifying and prioritizing capital-planning projects is the annual SCIP process. SCIP—first used in fiscal year 2010—is used not only to identify the capital required to meet VA's service and space needs but also to ensure that all project requests are centrally reviewed in an equitable and consistent way throughout the system. As part of the SCIP process, VA utilizes VAMC-level data from models (including VetPop and the Enrollee Health Care Projection Model) to determine "gaps" between the current state and the strategic capital goal. A SCIP "gap" is the difference between a current facility's square footage and its estimated future space needs. These data are updated and distributed annually to local VAMC staff for the development of plans for "closing" the gaps (i.e., reducing the gaps). The SCIP process calculates both positive (needs additional capacity) and negative (has excess capacity)

that the percentage of veterans' care at the VA and in the community should remain at present levels and another might assume that a larger percentage of future care will be provided in the community. According to VA officials, VA management decides which scenarios to use in determining estimates for a given year.

gaps between current and future space needs for 12 different categories of clinical and non-clinical space.[18] (See Figure. 1.)

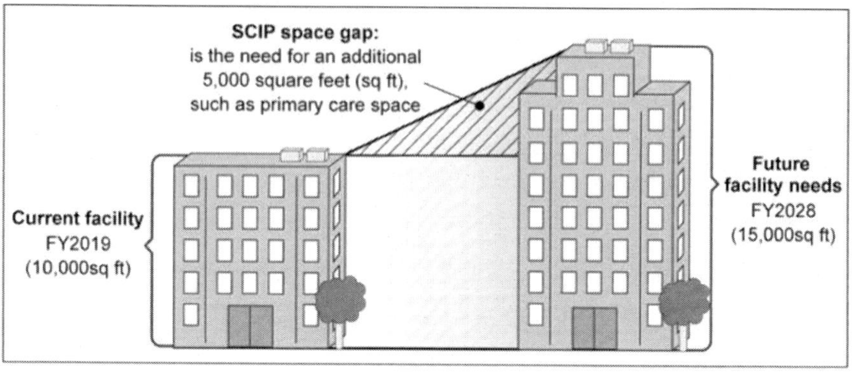

Source: GAO. | GAO-19-440.

Note: A SCIP "gap" is the difference between a current facility's square footage and its estimated future space needs.

Figure 1. Illustration of Strategic Capital Investment Planning (SCIP) "Gaps."

Capital Planning at the VISN and VAMC level

VA officials at the VISNs and VAMCs play a major role in the capital-planning process. Each VISN has a Capital Asset Manager and planning staff who are responsible for coordination and oversight of capital-planning activities and who work with the individual VAMCs' facility-planning officials. The capital-planning process includes several tools for the facility-planning officials to use, including the Enrollee Health Care Projection Model, the Health Systems Planning Application, and SCIP.[19]

---

[18] The 12 SCIP space gap categories are: (1) Acute Care: Acute Inpatient Medicine & Surgery; (2) Acute Care: Acute Special Programs; (3) Acute Care: Inpatient Mental Health; (4) Ambulatory Care: Ancillary/Diagnostic; (5) Ambulatory Care: Mental Health; (6) Ambulatory Care: Primary Care; (7) Ambulatory Care: Specialty Care; (8) Long Term Care: CLC/Hospice; (9) Non-Clinical Space: Administration; (10) Non-Clinical Space: Common/Vacant/Construction; (11) Non-Clinical Space: Research; and (12) Non-Clinical Space: Support.

[19] According to VA officials, the Health Systems Planning Application is a tool that facility planners can use to, among other things, help close their facility's gaps. These officials also

VA officials said that after the estimates from the Enrollee Health Care Projection model are prepared, facility-planning officials should undertake a health care planning process to better inform the SCIP process.

Through the SCIP process, VA encourages VAMC facility-planning officials to develop 10-year plans to address 95 percent of projected space needs, on an annual basis. According to VA, the department uses these plans to adapt its budget for infrastructure projects to changes in demographics that affect health care and benefits delivery. VAMC facility-planning officials then develop plans for the capital improvement projects that are expected to take place in the first year of the 10-year plan.

VA Assesses Trends in Veterans' Future Needs but Lacks a Process for Assessing Veterans' Changing Expectations

VA analyzes information about the needs of different veterans' groups and their demographic data to assess veterans' future needs for care. However, it lacks sufficient information to similarly assess how veterans' expectations for care may change over time. One of the VA officials responsible for the development of VA's strategic plan told us that veterans'

- needs refer to the care, benefits and support services veterans require to support their well-being and quality of life, and
- expectations refer to how veterans would like to receive the care, benefits, or support services that address their needs.[20]

Assessing needs: VA expects that demographic changes will affect both veterans' health care needs and expectations. Using the abovementioned definition, we found that VA assesses some aspects of

---

noted that the tool collects and displays additional data, including health care utilization projections from the Enrollee Health Care Projection Model and mapping tools.

[20] VA did not provide a definition of "needs" and "expectations" in its *FY 2018–2024 Strategic Plan*. However, VA provided these definitions when we asked them.

veterans' needs at the national level, a practice that may help VAMC facility planning officials avoid replication of efforts. For example, female veterans or those who served in specific military operations may have some similar health care needs regardless of where they are located, so it would not be necessary for multiple VAMCs to design and conduct separate studies of these populations. VA generates an overall depiction of how changes in veterans' demographics—including gender, service-connected disabilities, or age—will affect veterans' needs.[21] For example:

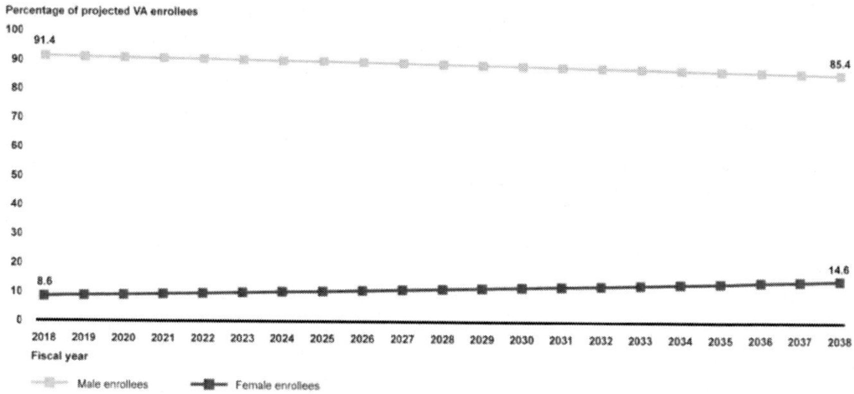

Source: GAO analysis of VA data. | GAO-19-440.

Note: These data are drawn from VA's Enrollee Health Care Projection Model from fiscal year 2017.

Figure 2. Department of Veterans Affairs' (VA) Projected Demographic Changes among VA Enrollees, by Gender (Fiscal Years 2018 through 2038).

- Gender: According to VA, female veterans of recent conflicts—such as the Gulf War and Operation Enduring Freedom, Operation Iraqi Freedom, and Operation New Dawn—make up over half of the female veterans who use VA services. Whereas the number of male enrolled veterans is estimated to decrease by almost 100,000 (8.03 million in fiscal year 2017 to 7.93 million by fiscal year 2027), the number of female enrolled veterans is expected to grow,

[21] VA's enrollment system for enrollees is based on a set of 8 priority groups to ensure health care benefits are readily available to all enrolled veterans.

increasing from 736,000 in fiscal year 2017 to 979,000 by fiscal year 2027. VA also estimates that the percentage of enrolled veterans who are female will continue to grow through fiscal year 2038. (See Figure 2.)

As the number of female veterans grows, VA estimates that there may be an increasing demand within VA for types of care specific to women, such as obstetrics.

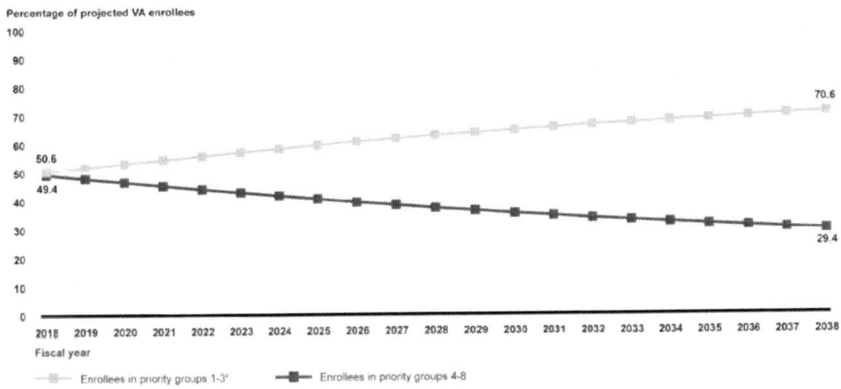

Source: GAO analysis of VA data. | GAO-19-440.

Notes: VA's enrollment system is based on 8 priority groups, with priority group 1 typically having the highest acuity or severity of disability.

These data are drawn from VA's Enrollee Health Care Projection Model from fiscal year 2017.

[a]VA combines priority groups 1-3 because enrollment in them is dependent on service-connected disabilities.

Figure 3. Department of Veterans Affairs' (VA) Projected Demographic Changes among VA Enrollees, by Priority Group (Fiscal Years 2018 through 2038).

- Service-Connected Disabilities: According to VA, veterans with service-connected disabilities rely on VA services to a significantly greater degree than do their counterparts without such disabilities. VA estimates that there will be an increase in the percentage of enrollees with service-connected disabilities in coming years. VA's enrollment system is based on 8 priority groups, and veterans' enrollment in priority groups 1 through 3 is based on service-connected disabilities.[22] The number and percentage of VA enrollees in groups 1-3 is currently about the same as those in groups 4-8 (those who do not have service-connected disabilities). As Figure 3 shows, however, VA estimates significant growth in the percentage of veterans who will be enrolled in priority groups 1-3 by fiscal year 2038.

According to VA, the growth in priority groups 1 through 3 is a key driver of demand for VA health care services. As enrollees transition into these groups, their reliance on VA health care significantly increases relative to those in other priority groups. Growth in these priority groups also affects specific VA services more than others, including home and community based care, outpatient mental-health services, and prosthetics.

- Age: VA also predicts that veterans' needs will change as younger cohorts enroll and older cohorts' reliance on VA services decreases as they become eligible for enrollment in the Medicare program.[23] This is in part because different cohorts have different needs. For example, VA officials told us that the cohort of veterans who entered military service immediately after the Vietnam War have a higher need for VA mental health services compared to other cohorts. According to VA, as older veterans' reliance on VA decreases, the needs of younger veterans of recent conflicts will have a larger effect on VA's health care services. Currently younger veterans make up a smaller proportion of VA enrollees than do older veteran cohorts. For example, at the end of fiscal year 2018, about 1.9-million VA enrollees were under the age of 45, about 2.7 million between the ages of 45– 64, and about 4.2 million aged 65 or older. However, VA estimates that the

[22] Priority group 1 is typically the most severely disabled (the highest acuity). There are also income requirements for certain veterans, including those who do not have a VA-rated service connected disability, which may influence which priority level they are placed in.

[23] According to VA, veterans' reliance on VA health care decreases beginning at age 65 as enrollees become eligible for Medicare coverage.

percentage of enrolled veterans who are between 45–64 will increase over the next 20 years. (See Figure 4.)

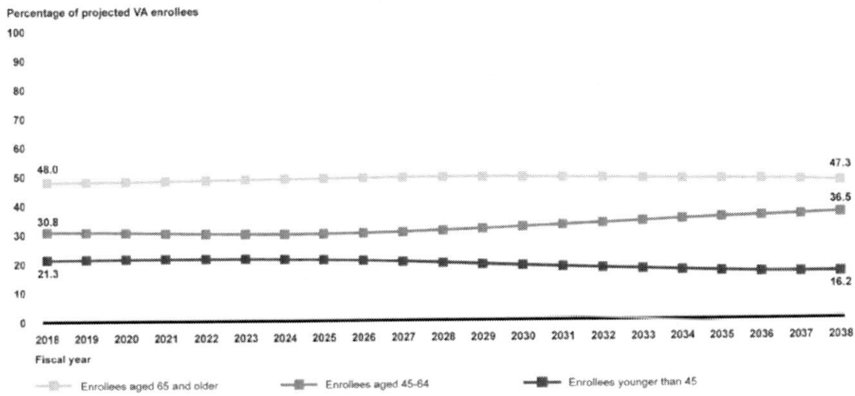

Source: GAO analysis of VA data. | GAO-19-440.

Note: These data are drawn from VA's Enrollee Health Care Projection Model from fiscal year 2017.

Figure 4. Department of Veterans Affairs' (VA) Projected Demographic Changes among VA Enrollees, by Age (Fiscal Years 2018 through 2038).

According to VA, reliance on VA health care tends to decrease beginning at age 65, as enrollees become eligible for Medicare coverage. Conversely, veterans may still rely on VA for certain types of services after age 65, and age drives growth in long-term care services and support, and other services generally not covered by private insurance or Medicare, such as hearing aids. VA officials told us that World War II enrollees are currently the highest users of long-term care services and support, with Vietnam Era enrollees projected to be an increased driver of demand for those services as they age.

Assessing expectations: While VA uses information about the needs of different groups in combination with demographic data to assess trends in veterans' future needs, it does not systematically collect data concerning how, if at all, demographic groups differ in their expectations for how they would like to receive care. Without this information, VA cannot provide VAMCs with national assessments of the expectations of different groups of veterans, as it does for their needs. VSOs, literature, and VAMC facility-planning officials have noted that demographic shifts may be driving changes in veterans' expectations for the care they receive from VA. According to literature and these VSOs and planning officials, these expectations can be relevant to facility planning and include:

- Convenience of care: Some younger veterans may prioritize "telehealth" more than older veterans.
- Privacy of care: Some younger veterans may expect to receive care in single-occupancy rooms rather than multi-occupancy. Additionally, female veterans may prefer to receive certain types of care in gender-separated environments.
- Scope of care: Some age groups may have a greater expectation for a holistic approach to their care, such as that promoted by VA's Whole Health initiative.[24]

VA officials told us that they learn about veterans' changing expectations through surveys and conversations with VSOs. We found, however, that the information VA collects through these efforts may be limited based on our review of VA's surveys and our discussions with five VSOs. Using the definition of veterans' expectations provided by VA, we analyzed the 14 surveys identified through our VA-coordinated review and determined that five surveys potentially included survey questions that specifically asked about veterans' expectations.[25] The amount of information that VA can ascertain about veterans' expectations from these five surveys, however, is limited because of the surveys' scope. Specifically:

Two of the five surveys were about specific services (i.e., retinal therapy and dermatology). Although each asked a question about the veteran's preference for receiving care via telehealth versus driving long distances, the surveys were focused primarily on veterans' satisfaction with

[24] The Whole Health initiative is intended to provide a holistic approach to health care that takes into consideration many life factors that can affects veterans' health, such as work environment, relationships, diet, and sleep patterns.

[25] The need to be able to link the responses to the respondent's demographic characteristics is key for being able to determine expectations for specific veterans' characteristics.

receiving this care via telehealth.[26] An official told us that VA has expanded this survey to additional services, but further review of the survey instrument showed that there are no longer any questions that specifically ask about veterans' expectations.

- The third survey—an annual survey of enrolled veterans' use of VA services—asks veterans about their experiences with VA health care, their reasons for choosing to seek care outside of VA, and the extent to which they use VA for their health care needs. However, our review found only one question that specifically asked about veterans' expectations, which asked the primary way veterans' expect to use VA in the future (e.g., as their primary source of health care, for prescriptions, etc.).[27]
- Finally, the last two surveys were administered in January and October 2015, respectively—and are no longer being conducted and only ask questions about five of the many types of VA health care.[28] These surveys were part of studies that asked veterans' about their expectations for how they receive primary or specialty care (i.e., appointment timeliness, type of provider, face-to-face vs. telehealth, distance traveled, etc.), and basic demographic characteristics, including gender, age, ethnicity, education, and health status.

Although VA officials told us they learn about veterans' expectations from discussions with VSOs, officials from three of the five VSOs we met with told us that they do not think that VA has a good understanding of the expectations of veterans as a whole, or certain groups of veterans. In addition, officials from the remaining two VSOs told us that they thought

---

26 The two surveys that focus on specific service lines are: VA's Teleretinal Patient Satisfaction Survey and VA's Tele-Dermatology Imaging Patient Satisfaction Survey.

27 VA's Survey of Veteran Enrollees' Health and Use of Health Care.

28 Specifically, the surveys asked questions about primary care in general and about four types of specialty care: orthopedics, oncology, endocrinology, and cardiology. These two surveys were part of VA's Primary Care Access Conjoint Study and VA's Specialty Care Conjoint Study, which have since been completed.

VA was collecting this information through veteran surveys. However, as we previously noted, the amount of information VA can ascertain on veterans' expectations from these surveys is limited.

VA's FY 2018–2024 Strategic Plan notes the need for VA to solicit veteran feedback and to continuously adapt benefits and care offerings to meet their changing needs and expectations. In addition, federal standards for internal control state that agencies should use quality information to achieve their objectives.[29] These standards specify that management identifies information requirements in an iterative and ongoing process and obtain relevant data from reliable internal and external sources in a timely manner. VA told us it uses surveys and interactions with VSOs to obtain information about veterans' satisfaction with aspects of their care. Our review of VA's surveys, however, found that VA may be limited in its ability to systematically assess trends in veterans' expectations due to the lack of explicit questions and measures of expectations for many types of VA health-care services—based on the definition of expectations provided by VA. Further, our discussions with VSOs suggest that VA may not be effectively collecting information from the VSOs on their members' expectations for care. Also, federal standards for internal control state that management should externally communicate necessary quality information. Management obtains quality information from external stakeholders—which in VA's case would be information from veterans—using established reporting lines that provide methods of communication that can flow down, across, up, and around the organizational structure.[30] This information includes significant matters relating to risks, changes, or issues that, in this case, affect VA's ability to meet its objective regarding veterans' changing expectations. We found that although VA understands how future shifts in veteran demographics will affect veterans' needs, VA lacks sufficient information about how these shifts will impact veterans' expectations over time. As a result, VA is at risk of:

---

[29] See GAO-14-704G.
[30] See GAO-14-704G.

- not accomplishing its strategic goal of meeting veterans' changing expectations by providing services in the way veterans want them provided, and
- VAMCs replicating each other's efforts to assess changes to veterans' expectations.

VA Has Made Addressing Veterans' Changing Needs and Expectations in Facility Planning a Priority but Lacks Instructions for Its Implementation

VA Established Meeting Veterans' Changing Needs and Expectations as a Strategic Goal but Did Not Provide VAMCs Instructions on How to Meet It

VA made soliciting and using veterans' changing needs and expectations a strategic goal. However, VA has not provided instruction to VAMC facility-planning officials on how to assess veterans' needs and expectations or incorporate them into their facility planning. For example, VA could identify certain resources or tools and direct VAMCs to use them. Federal standards for internal control state that management should internally communicate the necessary quality information to achieve the entity's objectives, i.e., implementing its strategic goal.[31]

During our site visits, it was clear that the facility-planning officials from the eight VAMCs we visited had not received instruction from VA on how to assess changes to veterans' needs and expectations. VA officials told us that they did not provide such instruction to the regional level (VISNs) or to the local level (VAMCs) because they believed most people understand what is meant by needs and expectations. However, we found during our site visits that there is a lack of consistent interpretation of what

[31] See GAO-14-704G.

these terms mean among facility-planning officials, a lack that was illustrated by the different approaches they used in assessing the changing needs and expectations of the veterans they serve. For example:

- Needs: In addition to using VA's health-care workload projection data, facility-planning officials at one VAMC we visited told us they use surveys and historical workload trends to assess changes to veterans' needs. Facility-planning officials at another VAMC told us they use surveys, town halls, focus groups, and meetings with VSOs and other stakeholders.
- Expectations: Facility-planning officials at one VAMC told us they use patient satisfaction data from surveys and information collected on patients' expectations in the private sector to assess changes to veterans' expectations. Facility-planning officials at another VAMC told us they use veterans' feedback, including information from VSOs and interactions between their facility's leadership with veterans.

Facility-planning officials' use of different approaches to assessing veterans' needs and expectations may not be concerning—different approaches may provide valuable information. However, without instruction on this from VA, VAMCs may miss out on opportunities to use other identified approaches for collecting this information as part of their facility planning efforts.

In addition, VA has not instructed facility planners on how to incorporate information about veterans' needs and expectations into facility planning. Although 71 percent of facility-planning officials responded in our survey that VA's expectations for incorporating veterans' demographics and the associated changes in their needs or expectations are moderately or very clear, about 87 percent responded that instructions from VA would be moderately or very useful. One survey respondent suggested that through such instruction, VA provide a "clear and concise direction" and another respondent suggested the instruction include "clearly established and communicated goals, objectives, and targets that are cascaded to VAMCs through VISNs." Without clear, internal communication explaining how it expects its stated goals to be achieved, VA cannot reasonably ensure that VAMCs' future facility plans are designed to meet veterans' changing needs and expectations.

VA Identified Foundational Health Services to Meet Some of Veterans' Expectations but Did Not Provide Clear Instruction on How to Implement the Effort

At the national level, VA selected a set of core medical services called "foundational health services," in part, according to VA officials, to meet veterans' expectations of consistent care offerings across VAMCs, and also to focus its resources on its highest priority services. However, based on our survey of VAMCs and discussions with selected facility-planning officials, we found that VA did not provide VAMC facility-planning officials with clear instruction on how to implement this effort. According to VA guidance, foundational health services focus on:

- the management of military disorders where care access is limited in the private market, such as a spinal cord injury and prosthetics, or
- care across the veterans' lifespan, including their primary care and geriatric care.[32]

VA's FY 2018–2024 Strategic Plan states "VA's emphasis on foundational services ensures veterans receive quality care for those conditions most attributed to military services and best provided by VA that optimizes their health, well-being, and quality of life." As for those services not defined as foundational (i.e., non-foundational services), a VA official responsible for leading VA's foundational services effort told us those services are still part of its health benefits package, but may or may

---

[32] VA's Memorandum on Foundational Services dated August 18, 2017.

not be provided at the VAMCs. VA's guidance further states that the decision to provide a non-foundational service is made locally, by individual VAMCs.

Department of Veterans Affairs' (VA) Foundational Health Services

According to VA's FY 2018–2024 Strategic Plan, VA's foundational health services are:

- Primary care,
- Urgent care,
- Mental health,
- Geriatrics and extended care,
- Rehabilitation,
- VA care coordination-such as case management,
- Post Deployment Health Services and War Related Illness and Injury Study Centers, and
- Pain management and opioid safety.

Source: VA's FY 2018–2024 Strategic Plan. | GAO-19-440.

A VA official responsible for leading VA's foundational services effort told us that foundational health services are the services that veterans can expect at each medical center. The list of these services is identified in VA guidance to VISNs and VAMCs. However, facility-planning officials at four of the VAMCs we visited during our site visits told us they did not know if the services VA specified were required to be delivered at each facility or if each facility could make changes to the list. Further, we found through our survey and site visits that VAMC facility-planning officials had defined different sets of foundational services for their facility. Specifically, approximately 10 percent of survey respondents said that their VAMC considers at least one VA-identified foundational health service to be non-foundational. In addition, officials from one of the VAMCs we visited told us they considered only six of VA's foundational health services to be foundational at their facility, while officials from another VAMC told us they only considered four (see Table 1).

Table 1. Examples of department of Veterans Affairs' (VA) medical centers with differing lists of foundational health services (February 2019)

VA's foundational health services	Foundational health services at one VA medical center (VAMC)	Foundational health services at another VAMC
Primary care	Yes	Yes
Urgent care	Yes	Yes
Mental health	Yes	Yes
Geriatrics and extended care	Yes	No
Rehabilitation	Yes	No
VA care coordination	Yes	No
Post Deployment Health Services and War Related Illness and Injury Study Centers	No	No
Pain management and opioid safety	No	Yes

Source: GAO analysis. | GAO-19-440.

Note: According to a VA official responsible for leading VA's foundational services effort, foundational health services are services that veterans can expect at each medical center.

Based on our survey of VAMCs and discussions with selected facility-planning officials, we found that VA did not provide clear instruction to facility planners on how to incorporate foundational and non-foundational health services into their facility planning.

- Foundational health services: In our survey, 42 percent of facility-planning officials reported that VA's expectations for how their facility should plan for foundational health services was "slightly" or "not at all" clear. A VA official responsible for leading VA's foundational services effort told us that the intent is for VA to provide all of the care for the foundational services at the VAMCs and not purchase any through community providers.[33] However, in

[33] This official told us that there may be some rare exceptions to providing foundational health services at the medical centers, but did not provide an example of a rare exception.

our discussions with facility-planning officials at five of the VAMCs we visited, it was clear that VA had not provided them with this information because they were unsure as to whether they could plan to obtain foundational services from community providers. Facility-planning officials at one of the VAMCs we met with told us their understanding was that some of the care for foundational health services could be provided by community providers. In contrast, facility-planning officials from another VAMC told us that their understanding was that none of the care for foundational health services could be provided by community providers.

- Non-foundational health services: Facility-planning officials from four of the VAMCs we visited told us they were unsure about how to plan for non-foundational health services and suggested a need for further clarification. This perspective was also shared by 12 facility planning officials who responded to our open-ended survey question that asked how, if at all, the information received from VA on the foundational services could be improved to help them prioritize their planning efforts.[34] For example, one survey respondent reported that "VA is not very clear on how to plan for these non-foundational services," and another wrote about the need to "understand what, if anything, is going to occur with non-foundational services."

In addition, facility-planning officials at five of the VAMCs we visited told us that they are unsure whether the foundational health services will continue to be a priority under current leadership—a concern that VHA officials also shared with us.[35] Accordingly, facility-planning officials told

[34] A total of 80 facility planning officials responded to this question. As the question was an open-ended survey question, respondents had the opportunity to list areas where they thought additional clarification was needed. In addition to suggesting further clarification on non-foundational health services, facility-planning officials also discussed needing clarification on what is included for each foundational service and explaining how the foundational services relate to the SCIP approval process.

[35] The foundational health services were established in late 2017 under the previous VA administration.

us that further instruction on the future implementation of foundational health services would be helpful. Specifically, in our survey, nearly four in five respondents (79 percent) reported that additional instruction from VA regarding incorporating foundational health services would be moderately or very useful. For example, one respondent noted that the instruction should be "concise, clear, and more explicit," and another that "communication [of foundational health services] needs to funnel down to the facilities better." Federal standards for internal control state that management should internally communicate the necessary quality information to achieve the entity's objectives.[36]

Although VA has issued guidance for foundational health services, it does not address how facility-planning officials should plan for foundational and non-foundational services. Foundational health services have important consequences for VA's facility planning, as VA's desire to prioritize which health care services should be offered consistently across VAMCs must be compatible with a constrained fiscal environment. However, based on our survey of VAMCs and discussions with selected facility-planning officials, we found that VA has not provided clear instruction regarding these services and has not told facility-planning officials whether the foundational health services remain a priority—guidance that would be an example of quality information. Moreover, VA increases the risk that it may not accomplish its goal of planning for the concept of foundational health services. This has further implications for meeting veterans' expectations of consistent care offerings across VAMCs and increases its risk that VAMCs are not focusing their resources on VA's highest priority services. Without this instruction, VAMC facility-planning officials may not successfully implement this effort through their facility planning—including the SCIP process, leaving VA at risk for VAMCs not focusing their resources on VA's highest priority services.

[36] See GAO-14-704G.

VAMC Facility Planners Are Concerned about VA's Process for Identifying Future Needs for Space in Facilities and Thus May Instead Rely on Locally Defined Priorities

VAMC Facility Planners Have Concerns about How SCIP's Estimated Space Needs Are Determined and Also Question the Estimates' Reliability and Usefulness

Although VA uses its SCIP process to identify facilities' future needs for space, we found that VAMC facility-planning officials have concerns about the SCIP estimates. VA annually provides VAMC facility-planning officials with 10-year estimates of future space needs for their facilities based on VA's estimates of veterans' future health-care needs. Specifically, VA uses facility-level utilization data from the Enrollee Health Care Projection Model to convert predicted utilization of VA health care services into future square footage needs with the SCIP process. However, in speaking to and surveying facility-planning officials at VAMCs, we found most do not fully understand the calculation of the SCIP space estimates, and to some extent questioned their reliability and usefulness.

- Calculation of SCIP's space estimates: VAMC facility-planning officials reported difficulties understanding how SCIP's space estimates are calculated from projected workload estimates. Specifically, 70 percent responded that this process was either slightly or not at all clear. In addition, 89 percent responded that further clarification about this process from VA would be moderately or very useful to their facility's planning efforts. Further, nearly 7 in 10 facility planner respondents (69 percent) responded that it was somewhat or very difficult to determine which of the 71 space categories (that they are more familiar with at their local level) to allocate the projected space changes from the

12 SCIP categories.[37] VA officials told us that they have included information about how these 71 space categories relate to the 12 SCIP space categories in a "crosswalk" they provided to the VAMCs. However, it does not include information on how to determine which of the 71 categories to allocate specific space needs to from a particular SCIP gap.

Of those respondents to GAO's survey who believed a particular Strategic Capital Investment Planning (SCIP) space gap—the difference between a current facility's square footage and estimated future space needs— was generally inaccurate in reflecting the projected space needs for the facility, 37 percent believed they actually needed less space than the estimate suggested. Nearly half of the survey's respondents (49 percent) noted that they did not know enough about how the space gaps were determined to understand what actually caused what they perceived as inaccuracies in the SCIP estimates. When asked to identify what they perceived as having contributed to the inaccuracies, facility planners most often responded that it was changing veteran needs and expectations or standards of care (56 percent) and inaccuracies with the actual demographic or workload estimates (54 percent).

Source: GAO survey of Department of Veterans Affairs' medical center facility-planning officials. | GAO-19-440.

- Reliability of SCIP space estimates: VAMC facility-planning officials believe that some SCIP space estimates do not accurately reflect the projected needs for their facilities, and some have reported large annual variations in the estimates. Specifically, facility planners at 72 percent of the facilities reported the estimated space needs for their facility as generally inaccurate in reflecting their facility's projected space needs for at least 1 of the 12 SCIP space categories.[38] Further, over half (51 percent) responded that estimates for 3 or more of the SCIP space categories were generally

[37] At the facility level, VAMC officials categorize their square footage into 71 space categories in the Capital Asset Inventory database. These 71 categories are more granular than SCIP's space categories, and each facility is required to annually validate that their space is accurately recorded.

[38] Across the 12 SCIP space categories, ratings of "generally inaccurate" range from 14 percent to 43 percent.

inaccurate in reflecting the projected space needs for their facility. The SCIP space categories most cited for inaccuracies were "Inpatient Mental Health," followed by "Administration" and "Acute Inpatient Medicine & Surgery."[39] For example, at one VAMC we visited, the SCIP process estimated an Inpatient Mental Health surplus of approximately 29,000 square feet. Facility-planning officials at the VAMC told us they disagreed with the estimate, saying that they anticipate growth in this area due to an increased focus on suicide prevention and a related VA policy change.[40] As such, they expect needing more space—not having a surplus of it. When asked about this particular concern, VA officials who oversee SCIP explained that the policy change took place after that year's SCIP space estimates had been calculated.[41] They acknowledged that there may also be specific instances where it is necessary to allow the facility planners to have some flexibility to deviate from the SCIP space estimates, and told us that facility-planning officials are encouraged to report any perceived inaccuracies to SCIP officials.[42]

Facility planning officials at two of the VAMCs we visited told us that they observed large variations in their facility's SCIP space estimates from year to year, which can make it difficult for planning purposes. In addition, one survey respondent noted that the "huge swings in gaps from year to year make it extremely challenging to put in valid projects for more than 1 or 2 years out." To better understand these views, we reviewed the 4 most-recent years of SCIP space estimates and found some annual variations.

---

[39] Nearly half of the respondents (43 percent) reported that they thought the "Inpatient Mental Health" SCIP space category was generally inaccurate in reflecting the projected needs for their facilities, followed by over one-third (34 percent) for the "Administration" category and (31 percent) for the "Acute Inpatient Medicine & Surgery" category.

[40] In 2018, VA identified suicide prevention as its highest clinical priority in its strategic plan for fiscal years 2018 through 2024 and, under a recent policy change allows for mental health treatment for veterans with other-than- honorable discharges.

[41] According to officials who oversee SCIP, the initial space projection was done in January 2017. The policy change was announced in July of 2017.

[42] SCIP officials told us that they did not receive feedback from this particular VAMC regarding this particular SCIP space estimate.

For example, for a given SCIP space category, we found that the median SCIP space estimates of what facilities would need in 10 years increased by 13 percent from the fiscal year 2019 SCIP space estimates to the fiscal year 2020 estimates (See Figure 5).

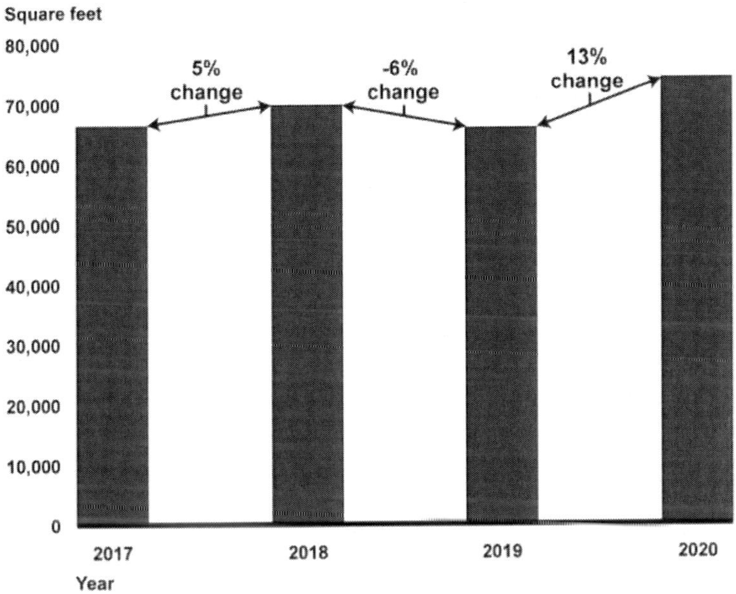

Note: The median SCIP space estimate represents the median projected 10-year space needs for a given SCIP space category.

Figure 5. Changes in the Median Estimated Space Need from the Strategic Capital Investment Planning (SCIP) Process, SCIP's Fiscal Year Estimates 2017, 2018, 2019, and 2020.

When we asked VA officials who oversee the Enrollee Health Care Projection Model and the SCIP process about these annual variations, they told us that the variations are primarily due to the Enrollee Health Care Projection Model's scenarios that VA applies to estimate how much veteran care will be outsourced to the community. VA officials who oversee the Enrollee Health Care Projection Model further stated that they communicate information about changes to the model annually to the VISNs and facilities through training classes. Officials at the VISNs we visited confirmed to us that VAMC planners are invited to these annual training classes and included on emails.

- Usefulness of SCIP space estimates: VAMC facility-planning officials also questioned the usefulness of the process for closing out SCIP gaps. Specifically, more than half of the facility planners (52 percent) responded that they thought the overall process of closing SCIP gaps was slightly or not at all useful to address the future needs and expectations of their local veteran population. Further, in order to close the SCIP space gaps on an annual basis, facility-planning officials at seven of the VAMCs we visited told us they frequently put in a project (that they may or may not actually have realistic plans to complete) in the out-years of the 10-year planning process called a "lump sum project." The facility planners told us they would use these projects to close whatever SCIP space gaps they did not think were correct or important to address.[43] For example, facility-planning officials at a VAMC with a reported space deficit for "common/vacant/construction" space in the hundreds of thousands of square feet said that they did not agree with this gap and had no intention of adding this much common space.[44] Nonetheless, they told us they added a lump-sum project to SCIP that suggests they would add hundreds of thousands of square feet of circulation space in order to close out the SCIP gap. Another facility planner echoed this sentiment by responding to the survey that the SCIP process "becomes an exercise of zeroing out numbers with lump sum out-year projects," and another noted that "gaps closed in out-year projects rarely come to fruition and certainly don't address current needs."

---

[43] In a January 2019 memorandum about the fiscal year 2021 SCIP process, VA notes that those out-year projects that are entered into SCIP must be projects that the facility has an intent to complete—and thus must be a "real and justifiable" project.

[44] For this particular VAMC, the facility planning officials told us that closing this particular SCIP space gap would require them to increase the current size of the entire facility by approximately 40 percent.

VA Facility Planners May Rely on Local Priorities Rather Than Using SCIP's Estimated Space Needs

Instead of using SCIP space estimates as a starting point to incorporate veterans' changing needs, VAMC facility planners may instead rely on local priorities, such as those identified by VAMC management or through feedback from local veterans. Specifically, due, in part, to their concerns with the SCIP process, facility-planning officials at five of the VAMCs we visited told us that instead of using the SCIP gaps to assist them in identifying what their future space needs are, they instead base these decisions on what they or their local management think are what the facility needs. For example, one VAMC we visited had—based on the SCIP process—an estimated 10-year surplus of approximately 4,000 square feet of inpatient mental health space. However, facility-planning officials at this VAMC told us that because their inpatient mental health beds are always at capacity, they are actually submitting projects to increase their space, and not decrease it.

> In reference to not always using the Strategic Capital Investment Planning (SCIP) space gaps—the difference between a facility's current square footage and estimated future space needs—as a starting point to determine needs and instead using local priorities, one survey respondent noted that: "The SCIP process often becomes fitting projects we need into filling the gaps," and "as with many centrally controlled processes, SCIP has become more of a 'how can we get our projects funded' tool than a 'this helps us plan' tool."

Source: GAO survey of Department of Veterans Affairs' medical center facility-planning officials. | GAO-19-440.

We also found that officials at VAMCs collect veterans' feedback through a variety of mechanisms and incorporate some of this information into their facility-planning efforts. For example, facility-planning officials from four of the VAMCs we visited told us that they obtain feedback from veterans on their needs and expectations through VA's national level satisfaction surveys, and incorporate this feedback into facility planning decisions. However, as we report above, the amount of information that

VA can ascertain about veterans' expectations from these surveys is limited.

Of the different methods available to collect feedback from veterans' on their needs and expectations, the method most cited by survey respondents was town halls (88 percent), followed by feedback from veterans' comments to providers/VA staff (85 percent), and then feedback from VSOs (80 percent).[45] Facility-planning officials use information from these efforts to inform their decisions. For example, facility-planning officials at one VAMC we visited told us that they coordinate with a particular VSO when considering changes to the Spinal Cord Injury or Polytrauma areas, as that VSO has knowledge of veterans' unique requirements in these areas. However, these methods for collecting information on veterans' needs and expectations are not consistent across VAMCs, making it even more important for VAMC facility planners to supplement their efforts with information on veterans' needs from the SCIP space estimates. For example, while town hall meetings can provide valuable feedback, they may not capture changing demographics and may only represent the most vocal veteran participants in attendance.

Federal standards for internal control state that management should use quality information to achieve the entity's objectives.[46] For example, this includes obtaining quality information through relevant data from reliable sources. Relevant data have a logical connection with the information requirements, and reliable data faithfully represent what it is purported to represent. Reliable sources include internal stakeholders. Further, the information needed is best identified in an iterative and ongoing process to address any risks identified in determining whether all the relevant

---

[45] In our survey of facility-planning officials, we asked which of the following sources of veteran's feedback they used as part of the facility planning process: VA-administered nationally representative surveys of veterans; VAMC- or VISN-administered surveys of only the veterans that go to your facilities or are in your VISN; town halls or other formal discussions with veterans; feedback from veterans' comments (e.g., comments to providers/VA staff, patient advocates, comment boxes, social media, etc.); feedback from VSOs, third party reports (e.g., VSO reports, RAND, etc.); or other sources. See appendix II for the survey questions.

[46] See GAO-14-704G.

information is obtained. VA expends significant effort on the SCIP process and expects VAMC facility-planning officials to use SCIP space estimates as starting points for incorporating veterans' changing needs into their facility planning, and then make local adjustments as necessary. However, VAMC facility-planning officials—citing confusion with the process and concerns about the reliability of some of the space gaps— are sometimes reluctant to use the SCIP estimates as the starting point for determining their future facility needs. These concerns can result in inconsistent use of SCIP estimates across the VAMCs and diminish the ability to equitably and systematically assess needs. Unless VA officials work with the VAMC facility-planning officials to understand and address their concerns with the SCIP process, VA may not have all the necessary information and the facility-planning officials may continue to miss out on an opportunity to incorporate veterans' changing needs. As a result, their planning may not sufficiently address veterans' changing needs and expectations. Moreover, VAMCs may spend time and resources to build something they may not need (resulting in excess capacity) or not focus these resources where additional capacity is needed (resulting in shortages).

CONCLUSION

VA's efforts to assist VAMCs in planning for shifts in veteran demographics, reflecting changing needs and expectations may only be partly successful and may lead to excess capacity in some facilities, and shortages in others. Over the next 10 to 20 years, an increasing percentage of veterans who are female and the aging of different wartime groups are just two of the many demographic shifts among veterans for which VA must prepare its medical facilities. Advance planning for the effects changes in veterans' needs and expectations will have on VAMCs' services and facilities is important as, for example, a construction project on a VAMC campus can take many years to complete. VA assesses how these shifts affect facility planning for veterans' needs but has not conducted an effort to assess the potential effects of veterans' changing expectations. Further, VA has not communicated to local VAMCs how to incorporate its strategic goal for addressing veterans' needs and expectations as part of their service and facility planning. Without a national effort to assess trends in veterans' changing expectations (as they have done for veterans' needs) or common instructions from VA, individual VAMCs may potentially replicate each other's efforts (e.g., in designing surveys) or use varying methods to assess how changes to their local veterans' population might alter their services and facilities. Moreover, without VA leadership fully explaining to VAMCs how to implement the concept of foundational health services, VA increases the risk that it may not accomplish its strategic goal of meeting veterans' expectations of consistent care across VAMCs, and that VAMCs are not focusing resources on high priority services. In addition, VAMC planning officials are not confident that the SCIP process is accurately converting veterans' future health-care needs into where appropriate space will be needed and at times are reluctant to use SCIP data as a starting point for decision-making. Without a systematic process in place for VA to identify and address concerns with the SCIP process, VAMC facility-planning officials may build space in facilities they will not need—or fail to build space they do need.

RECOMMENDATIONS FOR EXECUTIVE ACTION

To improve VA's ability to plan for and align its facilities with estimated changes to veterans' needs and expectations, we recommend that the Secretary of Veterans Affairs ensure the appropriate offices and administrations take the following four actions:

Develop and implement a process to assess veterans' changing expectations and disseminate this information to VAMCs. (Recommendation 1)

Instruct VAMCs on how to meet VA's strategic goal of incorporating veterans' changing needs and expectations into facility planning, such as by identifying certain resources or tools and directing VAMCs to use them. (Recommendation 2)

Provide additional instruction to VAMCs on how to incorporate the concept of foundational health services into facility planning. (Recommendation 3)

Systematically gather feedback from facility planners and address (as necessary) their concerns with the reliability of the SCIP process, including providing additional information on how SCIP's space estimates are derived. (Recommendation 4)

AGENCY COMMENTS AND OUR EVALUATION

We provided a draft of this chapter to VA for comment. Its written comments are reproduced in appendix III. VA concurred with our four recommendations. In response to our recommendation that VA develop and implement a process to assess veterans' changing expectations and disseminate this information to VAMCs, VA stated that it has already developed and implemented effective systems for obtaining veterans' input in facility planning. We have reviewed all materials that VA provided and continue to believe that they do not yet align with VA's definition of expectations. We will continue to monitor VA's efforts in this area and will close the recommendation when VA develops and implements a process to assess veterans' changing expectations, as defined by VA. Regarding our fourth recommendation, VA agreed to improve training for facility-planning officials. We still believe VA should also create a process for gathering and assessing legitimate concerns related to the SCIP process and make changes where appropriate. VA also provided technical comments, which we incorporated as appropriate, including a resulting clarification to our third recommendation. As a general comment, VA stated that we did not include information on its health care planning process, and we have added this information to our final report.

We are sending copies of this chapter to the Secretary of Veterans Affairs and the appropriate congressional committees.

Andrew Von Ah Director
Physical Infrastructure

Debra A. Draper Director
Health Care

APPENDIX I: OBJECTIVES, SCOPE, AND METHODOLOGY

This chapter examines: (1) the extent to which the Department of Veterans Affairs (VA) assesses trends in veterans' future needs and expectations; (2) VA's efforts to help VA medical centers (VAMC) address veterans' changing needs and expectations in planning VA's facilities; and (3) how VAMCs use VA's planning process for identifying future need for space in VA's facilities to address veterans' changing needs and expectations in facility planning.

To address these objectives, we reviewed relevant laws, regulations, policies, and VA's planning documents, including VA's FY 2018–2024 Strategic Plan.[47] We also interviewed officials from VA and VA's Veterans Health Administration (VHA) including from:

- VA's Central Office—including personnel from the Office of Asset Enterprise Management—and
- VHA's Central Office, including staff from its Office of Policy and Planning and Office of the Assistant Deputy Under Secretary for Health for Clinical Operations.[48]

In addition, we interviewed representatives from a broad range of national veterans' service organizations (VSO), including The American

[47] See Department of Veterans Affairs, *FY 2018–2024 Strategic Plan* (Washington, D.C.: February 2018).
[48] VHA operates VA's health care system, which includes VA medical centers and community-based outpatient clinics.

Legion, Vietnam Veterans of America, Disabled American Veterans, Iraq and Afghanistan Veterans of America, and Wounded Warrior Project.

To obtain local perspectives on the objectives, we surveyed those officials who are responsible for planning and making facility-planning decisions (hereafter referred to as "facility-planning officials") from all VAMCs. The survey addressed VA's efforts to assess trends in veterans' needs and expectations and incorporate the information in facility planning, and VA's SCIP process. We developed the survey based on our audit objectives, prior GAO work, and discussions with facility-planning officials. We pretested the survey with facility-planning officials at six VAMCs.[49] We administered our web-based survey between November 2018 and January 2019. One hundred thirty-seven individuals (of 139) responded to the survey (118 of the 119 facility-planning officials at single VAMCs and 19 of the 20 facility-planning officials that oversee multiple VAMCs), for an overall response rate of about 99 percent.[50] See appendix II for the survey questions and the summarized responses.

For more detailed information to supplement the survey, we visited a nongeneralizable sample of nine VAMCs located in four Veterans Integrated Service Networks (VISN) in August 2018 and September 2018.[51] (See Table 2.) We chose the nine VAMCs because they had relatively high needs for future space based on fiscal year 2019 data from VA's Strategic Capital Investment Planning (SCIP) process and

---

[49] We pretested the survey with VAMC facility-planning officials at the following six facilities that we selected based on future space needs (high and low) based on fiscal year 2020 data from VA's Strategic Capital Investment Planning (SCIP) process: (1-2) the VA Maryland Health Care System (Baltimore VAMC, Perry Point VAMC, and Loch Raven VAMC); (3) the Bay Pines VA Healthcare System (Bay Pines, Florida); (4) the James A. Haley Veterans' Hospital (Tampa, Florida); (5) the Cleveland VAMC (Cleveland, Ohio); (6) the Corporal Michael J. Crescenz VAMC (Philadelphia, Pennsylvania); and the Phoenix VA Health Care System (Phoenix, Arizona).

[50] We received responses from 137 of the 139 facility planning officials, representing 159 of the 162 VAMCs. Although there are 172 VAMCs, a VA official who oversees SCIP told us that VA combines several VAMC's SCIP space gap estimates as part of the SCIP planning process. As a result, VA attributes SCIP data to 162 VAMCs.

[51] VA organizes its system of care into regional networks called VISNs. Each VISN is responsible for managing and overseeing VA medical centers within a defined geographic area. We met with the planning officials at VISN 5 (District of Columbia, Maryland, Pennsylvania, Virginia, and West Virginia); VISN 6 (North Carolina and Virginia); VISN 8 (Florida, Georgia, Puerto Rico, and the U.S. Virgin Islands); and VISN 17 (Texas).

geographic proximity to each other. We conducted interviews with facility-planning officials at both the VISN and VAMC levels to discuss facility-planning resources, tools, and policies, and reviewed relevant documentation provided by these officials. At these nine VAMCs, we met with eight groups of facility-planning officials, because two of the VAMCs share a common set of facility-planning officials.[52] Results from our sample of site visits are not generalizable to all VISNs or VAMCs.

Table 2. Department of Veterans Affairs' (VA) Medical Centers Visited by GAO

VA medical center (VAMC)	Location	Veteran Integrated Service Network (VISN)
Baltimore VAMC	Baltimore, Maryland	VISN 5
Perry Point VAMC	Perry Point, Maryland	VISN 5
Hunter Holmes McGuire VAMC	Richmond, Virginia	VISN 6
Bay Pines VA Healthcare System	Bay Pines, Florida	VISN 8
Malcolm Randall VAMC	Gainesville, Florida	VISN 8
James A. Haley Veterans' Hospital	Tampa, Florida	VISN 8
Dallas VAMC	Dallas, Texas	VISN 17
Olin E. Teague Veterans' Medical Center	Temple, Texas	VISN 17
Audie L. Murphy VA Hospital	San Antonio, Texas	VISN 17

Source: GAO. | GAO-19-440.

Note: The Baltimore VAMC and Perry Point VAMC are part of the VA Maryland Healthcare System and, as a result, have the same facility-planning officials.

[52] Two of the VAMCs we visited, the Baltimore VAMC and Perry Point VAMC, are part of the VA Maryland Healthcare System and, as a result, have the same facility-planning officials. In many areas of the country, several medical centers and clinics may work together to offer services to area veterans as a health care system. According to VA, by sharing services between or among medical centers, the aim is for VHA to provide veterans easier access to advanced medical care closer to their homes.

To determine the extent to which VA assesses trends in veterans' needs and expectations, we reviewed documentation of the Enrollee Health Care Projection Model—a VA model for estimating the amount of resources VA needs to meet the expected demand for most of the health care services it provides—and interviewed officials at VHA's Office of Policy and Planning who oversee the model to discuss veteran population projections and trends.[53] We reviewed the model's documentation related to its purpose and structure and interviewed relevant officials, and determined that the data from the Enrollee Health Care Projection Model were sufficiently reliable for our audit objectives.[54] We also coordinated with VHA officials and relevant VAMC officials to identify 127 surveys that VA had been administering. In reviewing survey titles and coordinating with relevant survey points of contact, we narrowed down the 127 surveys to a list of 14 surveys by identifying those that could (1) potentially help VA understand veterans' needs and/or expectations in facility planning and (2) be attributed to different veteran population demographics (e.g., gender, age, race, etc.). We then reviewed these 14 survey instruments to determine the extent to which they included measures that specifically asked about veterans' expectations. Further, we compared VA's efforts to assess trends in veterans' needs and expectations to federal standards for internal control for use of quality information and relevant control activities.[55]

To identify what national efforts VA has initiated to help VAMCs address veterans' changing needs and expectations in facility planning, we reviewed VA documents, including its FY 2018–2024 Strategic Plan and relevant documentation about VA's foundational health services. We also interviewed officials from VHA's Office of Policy and Planning and Office of the Assistant Deputy Under Secretary for Health for Clinical Operations.

---

[53] The Enrollee Health Care Projection Model was developed in 1998 by VA and its consultant. It helps supports the development of VA's budget estimates for health care and informs strategic and capital planning.

[54] A review of the underlying assumptions of the Enrollee Health Care Projection Model and the accuracy of model projections was outside the scope of this review.

[55] GAO, *Standards for Internal Control in the Federal Government*, GAO-14-704G (Washington, D.C.: September 2014).

To obtain local perspectives on these efforts, we spoke with the facility-planning officials at each of the VISNs and VAMCs from our site visits and included questions about VA's instructions to VAMCs to implement these efforts in our national survey of facility planners. Further, we compared VA's national efforts to federal standards for internal control for communicating internally and relevant control activities.[56]

To determine how VAMCs use VA's process for identifying future facilities' space needs to address veterans' changing needs and expectations in facility planning, we spoke with the facility planning-officials at each of the VISNs and VAMCs from our site visits and included questions about the SCIP process (including its perceived reliability and usefulness) in our national survey of facility planners. Further, we analyzed SCIP data on estimates of facilities' needs for space in 10 years. Specifically, we analyzed variation in SCIP's estimate 10-year needs for space for all VAMCs across 4 years of SCIP data (SCIP fiscal years 2017, 2018, 2019, and 2020 estimates).[57] To assess the reliability of these data, we (1) performed electronic testing of relevant data elements; (2) reviewed existing information about the data and the system that produced them; and (3) interviewed agency officials knowledgeable about the data. We determined that these data were sufficiently reliable for presenting the estimates across the 4-year period. Further, we compared how VAMCs are using VA space estimates in their facility planning to federal standards for internal control for use of quality information and relevant control activities.[58]

We conducted this performance audit from April 2018 to June 2019 in accordance with generally accepted government auditing standards. Those standards require that we plan and perform the audit to obtain sufficient, appropriate evidence to provide a reasonable basis for our findings and conclusions based on our audit objectives. We believe that the evidence

---

[56] See GAO-14-704G.

[57] A given fiscal year's SCIP data are based on information collected 4 years prior. For example, SCIP data for fiscal year 2020 are based on information collected in fiscal year 2016, while SCIP data for fiscal year 2019 are based on information collected in fiscal year 2015.

[58] See GAO-14-704G.

obtained provides a reasonable basis for our findings and conclusions based on our audit objectives.

APPENDIX II: RESULTS OF GAO'S SURVEY OF DEPARTMENT OF VETERANS AFFAIRS' MEDICAL CENTER (VAMC) FACILITY-PLANNING OFFICIALS

In this appendix, we include all questions asked in our survey and results of responses to the closed-ended questions. Narrative answers to open-ended text questions are not displayed to prevent the identification of individual respondents. Percentages may not always sum to 100 percent because of rounding of decimal figures.

We administered our web-based survey between November 2018 and January 2019 to VAMC facility-planning officials. As noted in appendix I, 137 individuals representing 159 VAMCs responded to the survey (118 of the 119 facility-planning officials at single VAMCs and 19 of the 20 facility-planning officials that oversee multiple VAMCs), for an overall response rate of about 99 percent.[59] Because question-specific response rates varied in cases where individual questions were not answered, we show the total number of respondents for each question. Questions 11–22 ask about the facility planning officials' views on the accuracy of Strategic Capital Investment Planning (SCIP) process's 10-year projected space estimates for the officials' VAMC (or for each of the officials' VAMCs if they oversee multiple VAMCs). Of the 162 VAMCs' SCIP estimates that the survey asked about, facility-planning officials responded to the questions about their accuracy for 154 or 155 VAMCs (depending on the specific SCIP space category question).

[59] We received responses from 137 of the 139 facility-planning officials, representing 159 of the 162 VAMCs. Although there are 172 VAMCs, a VA official who oversees SCIP told us that VA combines several VAMC's SCIP space gap estimates as part of the SCIP planning process. As a result, VA attributes SCIP data to 162 VAMCs.

Facility Planning Resources

1. **Please indicate to what extent your facility uses the Health Systems Planning Application in its facility planning process. Then, please indicate if your facility has experienced any of the following issues with the Health Systems Planning Application.**

Use of the Health Systems Planning Application

Use to a large extent	Use to some extent	Use to a slight extent	Do not use	Total number of respondents
13%	36%	29%	21%	135

Notes: There were 137 possible respondents for this question. These percentages do not include those who did not respond to the question.

Problems identified with the Health Systems Planning Application

Relevancy	Accuracy	Completeness	"User friendly"	Other	No problems
19	25	22	29	32	43

Notes: There were 137 possible respondents for each question. Due to higher item non-response and the check-all-that-apply format, only counts of respondents who selected these answers are presented, rather than percentages.

If "Other" types of problems, please specify: *[text data intentionally not reported]*

2. **For each of the following types of data in the VHA Support Service Center Capital Assets portal/Pyramid, please indicate to what extent your facility uses each in its facility planning process. Then, please indicate if your facility has experienced any problems with these data.**

Use of data in the VHA Support Service Center Capital Assets portal/Pyramid

	Use to a large extent	Use to some extent	Use to a slight extent	Do not use	Total number of respondents
a. Enrollee Health Care Projection Model data within the VHA Support Service Center Capital Assets portal/Pyramid	59%	32%	4%	4%	136
b. Data other than the Enrollee Health Care Projection Model available in the VHA Support Service Center Capital Assets portal/Pyramid that is nationally collected and available at the facility level	56%	29%	10%	6%	136

Notes: There were 137 possible respondents for each question. These percentages do not include those who did not respond to the question.

Problems identified with the data in the VA Support Service Center Capital Assets portal/Pyramid

	Relevancy	Accessibility	Completeness	"User friendly"	Other	No Problems
a. Enrollee Health Care Projection Model data within the VHA Support Service Center Capital Assets portal/Pyramid	7	31	6	33	28	55
b. Data other than the Enrollee Health Care Projection Model available in the VHA Support Service Center Capital Assets portal/Pyramid that is nationally collected and available at the facility level	8	17	11	28	18	59

Notes: There were 137 possible respondents for each question. Due to higher item non-response and the check-all-that-apply format, only counts of respondents who selected these answers are presented, rather than percentages.

If "Other" types of problems, please specify: *[text data intentionally not reported]*

3. **For each of the following sources of veteran feedback, please indicate to what extent your facility uses each in its facility planning process. Then, please indicate if your facility has experienced any of the following problems with the sources of veteran feedback. (Please respond for each source of feedback.)**

Use of sources of veteran feedback

	Use to a large extent	Use to some extent	Use to a slight extent	Do not use	Don't know	Total number of respondents
a. VA-administered nationally representative surveys of veterans	34%	37%	15%	8%	6%	135
b. VAMC- or Veterans Integrated Service Network (VISN)-administered surveys of only the veterans that go to your facilities or are in your VISN	27%	32%	10%	18%	13%	135
c. Town halls or other formal discussions with veterans	56%	33%	10%	1%	1%	135
d. Feedback from veterans' comments (e.g., comments to providers/VA staff, patient advocates, comment boxes, social media, etc.)	58%	26%	12%	3%	1%	136

e. Feedback from veterans service organizations (VSO)s	45%	35%	17%	1%	1%	135
f. Third party reports (e.g., VSO reports, RAND, etc.)	13%	43%	21%	11%	12%	134

Notes: There were 137 possible respondents for each question. These percentages do not include those who did not respond to the question.

3g. Does your facility use any other sources of veteran feedback that are not listed above?

Yes	No	Total number of respondents
45%	55%	136

Notes: There were 137 possible respondents for each question. These percentages do not include those who did not respond to the question.

If "Yes", please describe the other sources: *[text data intentionally not reported]*

Problems identified with different sources of veteran feedback

	Relevancy	Accessibility	Not conducted	Other	No problems
a. VA-administered nationally representative surveys of veterans	20	19	NA	35	60
b. VAMC- or VISN-administered surveys of only the veterans that go to your facilities or are in your VISN	7	6	7	17	73
c. Town halls or other formal discussions with veterans	21	NA	0	21	83
d. Feedback from veterans' comments (e.g., comments to providers/VA staff, patient advocates, comment boxes, social media, etc.)	16	NA	0	17	85
e. Feedback from VSOs	13	NA	1	15	85
f. Third party reports (e.g., VSO reports, RAND, etc.)	11	13	NA	16	65

Notes: There were 137 possible respondents for each question. Due to higher item non-response and the check-all-that-apply format, only counts of respondents who selected these answers are presented, rather than percentages.

If "Other" types of problems, please specify: *[text data intentionally not reported]*

Facility Planning and Veterans' Changing Demographics

4. How clear, if at all, are VA's expectations regarding how to incorporate veterans' changing demographics and the associated changes in their needs or expectations into your facility planning?

Very clear	Moderately clear	Slightly clear	Not at all clear	Total number of respondents
29%	41%	18%	12%	136

Notes: There were 137 possible respondents for each question. These percentages do not include those who did not respond to the question.

5. **How useful, if at all, would instructions from VA regarding how to incorporate veterans' changing needs or expectations into facility planning be to your facility?**

Very useful	Moderately useful	Slightly useful	Not at all useful	Total number of respondents
61%	26%	11%	2%	137

Notes: There were 137 possible respondents for each question. These percentages do not include those who did not respond to the question.

VA's Foundational Health Services

6. **Facility foundational health services and VA's list of foundational health services**

	Yes	No	Don't know	Total number of respondents
a. Does your facility consider any additional services, not included on VA's list, to be foundational?	57%	37%	6%	137
b. Does your facility consider any services (1 or more) included on VA's list to be not foundational?	10%	86%	4%	136

Notes: There were 137 possible respondents for each question. These percentages do not include those who did not respond to the question.

7. **To what extent, if at all, does your facility plan for foundational services (as identified either by VA or your facility) differently from non-foundational services as part of its facility planning process?**

To a large extent	To some extent	To a slight extent	Not at all	Total number of respondents
33%	47%	12%	9%	137

Notes: There were 137 possible respondents for each question. These percentages do not include those who did not respond to the question.

8. **How clear, if at all, are VA's expectations for how your facility should plan for foundational services (as identified either by VA or your facility) versus non-foundational services?**

Very clear	Moderately clear	Slightly clear	Not at all clear	Total number of respondents
24%	35%	24%	18%	136

Notes: There were 137 possible respondents for each question. These percentages do not include those who did not respond to the question.

9. **How useful, if at all, would additional instruction from VA regarding incorporating foundational services (as identified either by VA or your facility) into facility planning be for your facility?**

Very useful	Moderately useful	Slightly useful	Not at all useful	Total number of respondents
51%	28%	17%	4%	135

Notes: There were 137 possible respondents for each question. These percentages do not include those who did not respond to the question.

10. **To what extent, if at all, has the information you have received from VA regarding planning for foundational services (as identified either by VA or your facility) helped you to prioritize your facility planning efforts?**

To a large extent	To some extent	To a slight extent	Not at all	Total number of respondents
27%	44%	21%	8%	137

Notes: There were 137 possible respondents for each question. These percentages do not include those who did not respond to the question.

10a. **How, if at all, could the information you received from VA on the foundational services (as identified either by VA or your facility) be improved to help you prioritize your facility planning efforts?**

[text data intentionally not reported]

VA's SCIP Process Space Gaps

11a – 22a: As you were closing out your fiscal year (FY) 2020 SCIP space gaps, was this projection generally accurate or generally inaccurate at reflecting the projected needs for your facility?

	Generally accurate	Generally inaccurate	Don't know	Total number of respondents
11a. Acute Care: Acute Inpatient Medicine & Surgery	55%	31%	14%	154
12a. Acute Care: Acute Special Programs	71%	14%	15%	154
13a. Acute Care: Inpatient Mental Health	43%	43%	14%	154
14a. Ambulatory Care: Ancillary/Diagnostic	61%	25%	14%	154
15a. Ambulatory Care: Mental Health	57%	30%	13%	155
16a. Ambulatory Care: Primary Care	68%	22%	10%	155
17a. Ambulatory Care: Specialty Care	66%	20%	14%	154
18a. Long Term Care: CLC/Hospice	57%	28%	15%	155
19a. Non-Clinical Space: Administration	50%	34%	16%	154
20a. Non-Clinical Space: Common/Vacant/Construction	56%	23%	20%	154
21a. Non-Clinical Space: Research	65%	20%	15%	154
22a. Non-Clinical Space: Support	63%	21%	16%	155

Notes: These questions were asked at the facility level, and as a result, there were 159 possible respondents for each question. These percentages do not include those who did not respond to the question. Although there were 137 possible survey respondents, 19 of the possible survey respondents were facility-planning officials for more than one VAMC.

11b – 22b: If "Generally inaccurate:" Which of the following best describes any inaccuracies of the projected space gap for this category?

	More space needed	Less space needed	Total number of respondents
11b. Acute Care: Acute Inpatient Medicine & Surgery	67%	33%	49
12b. Acute Care: Acute Special Programs	86%	14%	21
13b. Acute Care: Inpatient Mental Health	69%	31%	65
14b. Ambulatory Care: Ancillary/Diagnostic	42%	58%	38
15b. Ambulatory Care: Mental Health	63%	37%	46
16b. Ambulatory Care: Primary Care	82%	18%	33
17b. Ambulatory Care: Specialty Care	40%	60%	30
18b. Long Term Care: CLC/Hospice	62%	38%	42
19b. Non-Clinical Space: Administration	88%	12%	52
20b. Non-Clinical Space: Common/Vacant/Construction	38%	62%	37
21b. Non-Clinical Space: Research	62%	38%	29
22b. Non-Clinical Space: Support	53%	47%	32

Notes: These questions were asked at the facility level, and as a result, there were 159 possible respondents for each question. These percentages do not include those who did not respond to the question. Although there were 137 possible survey respondents, 19 of the possible survey respondents were facility-planning officials for more than one VAMC.

Overall SCIP Questions

23. When closing each of 12 SCIP space gaps, how easy or difficult is it to determine which of the 71 Capital Asset Inventory categories to allocate the changes in space to?

Very easy	Somewhat easy	Somewhat difficult	Very difficult	Total number of respondents
8%	23%	56%	14%	133

Notes: There were 137 possible respondents for each question. These percentages do not include those who did not respond to the question.

24. Do any of the following issues contribute to inaccuracies with the SCIP space gaps?

	Yes	No	Don't know	Total number of respondents
a. Inaccuracies in our facility's Capital Asset Inventory	43%	40%	17%	136
b. Inaccuracies with projections (e.g., demographics, workload, etc.)	54%	21%	24%	136
c. Inaccuracies with the translation of the projections into square footage	49%	24%	27%	136
d. Inaccuracies due to changing veteran needs and expectations and/or standards of care	56%	21%	22%	135
e. Don't know enough about how the gap was calculated to understand what caused the error	49%	33%	19%	135
f. Other	42%	27%	31%	95

Notes: There were 137 possible respondents for each question. These percentages do not include those who did not respond to the question.

If "Yes" for "Other", describe any additional issues regarding the accuracy of SCIP space gaps below: *[text data intentionally not reported]*

25. How clear, if at all, is the process that VA uses to translate projected utilization into square footage for the SCIP space gap projections for the 12 categories?

Very clear	Moderately clear	Slightly clear	Not at all clear	Total number of respondents
8%	22%	40%	29%	136

Notes: There were 137 possible respondents for each question. These percentages do not include those who did not respond to the question.

26. How useful, if at all, would further clarification about this process from VA be to your facility planning efforts?

Very useful	Moderately useful	Slightly useful	Not at all useful	Total number of respondents
65%	25%	8%	2%	133

Notes: There were 137 possible respondents for each question. These percentages do not include those who did not respond to the question.

27. As part of your facility planning, how useful do you find the overall process of closing SCIP gaps in order to address future needs and expectations of your local veteran population?

Very useful	Moderately useful	Slightly useful	Not at all useful	Total number of respondents
19%	29%	38%	15%	136

Notes: There were 137 possible respondents for each question. These percentages do not include those who did not respond to the question.

27a. What was your reasoning for how you answered about the usefulness of the overall process of closing out SCIP gaps?

[text data intentionally not reported]

28. VAMC officials are required to annually close out all of their SCIP gaps by submitting projects based on a 10-year planning cycle through SCIP. How useful is it to your facility to submit projects across a full 10-year SCIP planning cycle?

Very useful	Moderately useful	Slightly useful	Not at all useful	Total number of respondents
13%	25%	40%	21%	136

Notes: There were 137 possible respondents for each question. These percentages do not include those who did not respond to the question.

28a. What was your reasoning for how you answered about the usefulness of submitting projects across a full 10-year SCIP planning cycle?

[text data intentionally not reported]

29. What, if anything, would help you better plan for the changing needs and expectations of veterans?

[text data intentionally not reported]

APPENDIX III: COMMENTS FROM THE DEPARTMENT OF VETERANS AFFAIRS

THE SECRETARY OF VETERANS AFFAIRS
WASHINGTON

May 22, 2019

Mr. Andrew Von Ah
Director
Physical Infrastructure Issues
U.S. Government Accountability Office
441 G Street, NW
Washington, DC 20548

Dear Mr. Von Ah:

The Department of Veterans Affairs (VA) has reviewed the Government Accountability Office (GAO) draft report: ***VA REAL PROPERTY: Improvements in Facility Planning Needed to Ensure VA Meets Changes in Veterans' Needs and Expectations*** (GAO-19-440).

The enclosure contains the actions that VA will take to address the draft report recommendations.

VA appreciates the opportunity to comment on your draft report.

Sincerely,

Robert L. Wilkie

THE SECRETARY OF VETERANS AFFAIRS
WASHINGTON

May 22, 2019

Ms. Debra A. Draper
Director, Health Care
U.S. Government Accountability Office
441 G Street, NW
Washington, DC 20548

Dear Ms. Draper:

The Department of Veterans Affairs (VA) has reviewed the Government Accountability Office (GAO) draft report: ***VA REAL PROPERTY: Improvements in Facility Planning Needed to Ensure VA Meets Changes in Veterans' Needs and Expectations*** (GAO-19-440).

The enclosure contains the actions that VA will take to address the draft report recommendations.

VA appreciates the opportunity to comment on your draft report.

Sincerely,

Robert L. Wilkie

Department of Veterans Affairs (VA) Comments to
Government Accountability Office (GAO) Draft Report
VA REAL PROPERTY: Improvements in Facility Planning Needed to Ensure VA Meets Changes in Veterans Needs and Expectations
(GAO-19-440)

General Comment:

As discussed with GAO at the exit conference, the report does not address the health care planning process that the Veterans Health Administration (VHA) utilizes. That health care planning process is the missing step for facility planners to develop both capital and non-capital solutions to address the workload projections that are derived from the Enrollee Health Care Projection Model (EHCPM). That health care planning process is designed to occur after the EHCPM estimates are generated--but before the Strategic Capital Investment Plan (SCIP) process is initiated--to better inform the inputs the facility will need to put into SCIP. While the inclusion of this health care planning process may not change the recommendations GAO has made, it would ensure the process VA utilizes is properly and accurately explained in the report.

Recommendation 1: Develop and implement a consistent process to assess veterans' changing expectations and disseminate this information to VAMCs.

VA Comment: Concur. VHA has already developed and implemented effective systems for obtaining Veterans' input in facility planning. Depending on the project, VHA uses multiple modalities for obtaining this input, such as: townhalls, focus groups, demographic based surveys, Veterans signals (Vsignals), data from the Office of Policy and Planning, and general public comment. Vsignals allows each service such as pharmacy, imaging, or even location such as a Community Based Outpatient Clinic to see in real time the feedback that their Veterans have given them. This means that each team can review their performance routinely and make quick corrective actions based on that feedback. They have access to the right information at the right time. Veterans Integrated Service Networks (VISN) and VA Medical Centers (VAMC) use these mechanisms to ensure local needs and expectations are understood and addressed in facility planning. VHA uses an electronic system to collect and store Veterans' input from feedback surveys. VA feels this system is effective and consistent and has been in place for some time. Should VHA determine that a facility planning requirement gained from the input systems be implemented nationwide, it would be incorporated into national standards. For example, standard construction specifications and facility design are used throughout VA. VHA finds actions on this recommendation to be completed and requests GAO consider closure of this recommendation.
Status: Complete

Recommendation 2: Instruct VAMCs on how to meet VA's strategic goal of incorporating veterans' changing needs and expectations into facility planning, such as identifying certain resources or tools and directing VAMCs to use them.

VA Comment: Concur. VHA's Office of Capital Asset Management Engineering and Support (OCAMES) agrees that refreshing the requirement to use the Vsignals system data to assist in planning and updates will help ensure Veterans input is incorporated where appropriate. OCAMES will provide guidance to VAMCs in conjunction with the Office of Asset Enterprise Management's annual call memo for the SCIP program to remind VISNs and VAMCs to ensure that Vsignals data is used in preparation for SCIP planning process.
Target Completion Date: September 2019

Recommendation 3: Assess the extent to which its concept of foundational services is still a priority and communicate the results to VAMCs, and if still a priority, include additional instruction to VAMCs on how to incorporate into facility planning.

VA Comment: Concur. VHA appreciates GAO's finding that VAMCs have variable understanding of national guidance on foundational services. We define our vision for a modernized VHA as "Consistent delivery of excellent-quality care and customer service for every patient, every time." Our plan for modernization encompasses ten lanes of effort that, when taken together, enable VHA to function as an integrated high reliability organization. The ten lanes of effort are:

- Commit to Zero Harm
- VA MISSION Act: Improve Access to Care
- Engaging Veterans in Lifelong Health, Well-being, and Resilience
- Reduce Unwarranted Variation Across Integrated Clinical and Operational Service Lines
- Streamline VHA Central Office
- Revise Governance Processes and Align Decision Rights
- Develop Responsive Shared Services
- Modernize Electronic Health Records
- Transform Financial Management System
- Transform Supply Chain

The Office of the Deputy Under Secretary for Health for Operations and Management will clarify prior guidance on foundational services for Medical Centers. VHA looks forward to improving Veterans health care through modernization.
Target Completion Date: June 2019

Recommendation 4: Increase the value and reliability of the Strategic Capital Investment Planning (SCIP) process for facility planners by systematically gathering feedback from facility planners and addressing their concerns with the SCIP process (as necessary), including providing additional information on how SCIP space estimates are derived.

VA Comment: Concur. VA's training for the SCIP process will be modified to include additional explanation on how SCIP space estimates are derived. Training will specify how both clinical and non-clinical space is generated and how it relates to projected station workloads. Training will also specify what is expected in terms of gap closure for both clinical and non-clinical space estimates.

Additionally, VA will develop a survey to be released after training to ensure that users understand key concepts. It will also survey if users would like additional training on the SCIP Automation tool, how their gaps (including space estimates) are generated, and other topics related to the SCIP process. Staff will use the results of those surveys to either schedule individual or small-group training to address those users concerns and/or develop improvements to the SCIP process as needed.
Target Completion Date: May 2020

CONTENTS OF EARLIER VOLUMES

Key Government Reports. Volume 24: June 2019

Key Government Reports. Volume 23: June 2019

INDEX

A

B

C

D

E

F

G

N

O

P

V

W